The Play of Children: Current Theory and Research

Contributions to Human Development

Vol. 6

Series Editor

J.A. Meacham, Buffalo, N.Y.

S. Karger · Basel · München · Paris · London · New York · Sydney

The Play of Children: Current Theory and Research

Volume Editors
D.J. Pepler, Mississauga, Ont.
K.H. Rubin, Waterloo, Ont.

1 figure and 11 tables, 1982

S. Karger · Basel · München · Paris · London · New York · Sydney

Contributions to Human Development

Vol. 4: Issekutz Wolsky, M. de, and Wolsky, A., New York, N.Y.
The Mechanism of Evolution: A New Look at Old Ideas
VIII + 160 p., 3 fig., 3 tab., 1976. ISBN 3-8055-2347-5

Vol. 5: Social Development in Youth: Structure and Content
Meacham, J.A., Buffalo, N.Y., and Santilli, N.R., Washington, D.C. (eds.)
XII + 188 p., 2 fig., 18 tab., 1981. ISBN 3-8055-2868-X

National Library of Medicine, Cataloging in Publication
The Play of children: current theory and research/
volume editors, D.J. Pepler, K.H. Rubin. – Basel; New York: Karger, 1982.
(Contributions to human development; v. 6)
1. Play and Playthings I. Pepler, D.J. II. Rubin, K.H. III. Series
W1 C0778S v. 6 [WS 105.5.P5 P722]
ISBN 3-8055-3540-6

Printed in Switzerland by Tanner & Bosshardt AG, Basel
ISBN 3-8055-3540-6

Contents

Pretense Play in Early Childhood

Ecological Influences on Children's Play

To our first playmates, our parents:
Jane Pepler
Sunny and Jerry Rubin

Preface

In this volume we have attempted to provide the psychologist and educator interested in children's play with an overview of the major theoretical and research-based issues dominating the field today. Consequently the contributions concern such wide-ranging topics as the early theoretical roots of contemporary play research and the definition of play. Moreover, different types of children's play are considered at various points in infancy and childhood. Finally, critiques of extant research and suggestions for future directions have been formally included as separate chapter contributions.

The chapter contributions have been written by many of the leading figures in the study of children's play. We thank them for their efforts. We would also like to thank *Andrew German* and *Amy and Joshua Rubin*, our children, for providing us with first-hand insights into what children's play is all about.

Debra J. Pepler
Kenneth H. Rubin

Pg. 1-32

Contr. hum. Dev., vol. 6, pp. 1–3 (Karger, Basel 1982)

Introduction

The study of play in childhood is most definitely following an accelerative path. In the past 5 years or so more than 20 research-based books have been published in the area of children's play [*Sutton-Smith*, 1982]. Moreover, in a recent *Handbook of Child Psychology* (chapter on play), *Rubin* et al. [1982] cite approximately 450 different journal articles, books and convention presentations concerning the psychological aspects of children's play of which 20% were dated between 1970 and 1974, 38% between 1975 and 1979, and 14% after 1980. Given the exhaustive literature review in the *Handbook* chapter, it is interesting to discover that over 50% of the extant writings have been produced after 1975.

Why has there been such a sudden upswing in the psychological study of play? We think it may be related to a rediscovery of how a phenomenon once thought to be developmentally trivial and psychologically irrelevant [*Montessori*, 1973; *Schlosberg*, 1947] actually can play a major role in development. In recent years the Piagetian [1962] view that play reflects 'pure assimilation and egocentrism' has been translated into the view that play provides a psychometrically useful mirror of the development of symbolic representation [*Rubin* et al., 1982; *Rubin and Pepler*, 1980]. Further, play is viewed as consolidating and strengthening newly learned schemas [*Fein*, 1979; *Saltz*, 1980] and as directly causing advances in cognitive, social and social-cognitive development [*Saltz and Brodie*, this volume].

Having provided a rationale for why there is a prevalent belief that play is worth studying, the question to be asked is: 'What is there left to say about the phenomenon?' The answer may be drawn from the *Handbook* chapter in which *Rubin* et al. [1982] indicate countless areas and issues that remain to be studied and/or addressed. Many of these areas and issues are examined in this volume. In the opening chapter, *Rubin* provides a picture of continuity between the classical play theories (i.e., surplus energy, practice and recapitulation theories) and contemporary theory and research. He indicates that many contemporary issues concerning the developmental nature of play and the relations between different forms of play (e.g., pretense activity) and other developmental variables (e.g., creativity, problem-solving) were discussed in the early writings of *Spencer* [1873], *Groos* [1901] and *Bühler* [1928], among others. This overview of early theory and research thus provides a historical framework for the contemporary issues addressed in the remaining chapters.

Both *Vandenberg* and *Matthews and Matthews* address the problem of defining play. *Vandenberg* asks whether it is necessary to precisely define a psychological phenomenon to study it. *Matthews and Matthews* present an interesting methodological twist on how one particular form of play, pretense, might be reliably observed.

Another issue addressed by contemporary play researchers [*Fein*, 1975; *Wolf and Gardner*, 1979] concerns correlates and individual differences of early symbolic representational skills in infancy and toddlerhood. *McCune-Nicolich and Bruskin* examine the premise that a connection exists between symbolic play and language development. They present data that suggest two parallel structures in the development of symbolic play and language: (a) the transition to combinations and (b) the development of hierarchical symbolic structures allowing behaviors in play and language to be guided by prior mental acts. *Wolf and Grollman* present an interesting individual differences approach to the development of symbolic thinking. Based on a longitudinal study, they identify two types of pretense players, those who appear to prefer object-independent fantasy play and those who prefer object-dependent transformational play. They suggest that these contrasting preferences represent styles of play or differing orientations as opposed to a developmentally ordered progression. Their work raises questions about the correlations between these patterns of interest evidenced in pretense play and skills outside the realm of play.

Another major issue concerns the connection between different forms of play and the development of problem-solving skills. Several theorists [*Bruner*, 1972; *Groos*, 1901] have suggested that play facilitates both convergent and divergent problem-solving. *Pepler* examines the theoretical bases and empirical evidence concerning correlational and causal connections between play and divergent thinking or creativity. *Cheyne* critically evaluates extant research in which investigators attempt to demonstrate a causal link between play and convergent problem-solving.

Psychologists and educators alike have also speculated that pretense activities play a causal role in the development of social, cognitive and social-cognitive skills. The chapters by *Saltz and Brodie* and *Brainerd* both critically examine the causal link between pretense play training and social, cognitive and social-cognitive development. Interestingly, they come to quite different conclusions. *Saltz and Brodie* tend to view the developmental potential of pretense play far more positively than *Brainerd*, who questions the validity of play training for cognitive development.

A final issue addressed in this volume concerns ecological influences on children's play. That is, how does the classroom setting or general environmental venue influence the play of children? This is an important area of play research, since it might enable us to make predictions about children's behaviors within given environments and thereby allow the creation of play environments that elicit certain valued play behaviors. *Johnson and Ershler* review the research on the effects that different preschool programs have on children's play. As an example, they discuss their own study comparing the play of children in low-structure and high-structure preschool programs. In the final chapter, *Darvill* presents a critique of the research concerning the ecological influences on play and suggests future research directions.

References

Bruner, J.S.: The nature and uses of immaturity. Am. Psychol. *27:* 687–708 (1972).
Bühler, C.: Kindheit und Jugend (Hirzel, Leipzig 1928).
Fein, G.: A transformational analysis of pretending. Devl Psychol. *11:* 291–296 (1975).
Fein, G.: Play and the acquisition of symbols; in Katz, Current topics in early childhood education (Ablex, Norwood, N.J. 1979).
Groos, K.: The play of man (Appleton, New York 1901).
Montessori, M.: The Montessori method (Bentley, Cambridge, Mass. 1973).
Piaget, J.: Play, dreams and imitation in childhood (Norton, New York 1962).
Rubin, K.H.; Fein, G.; Vandenberg, B.: Play; in Hetherington, Handbook of child psychology: social development; 4th ed. (Wiley, New York, in press 1982).
Rubin, K.H.; Pepler, D.J.: The relationship of child's play to social-cognitive development; in Foot, Chapman, Smith, Friendship and childhood relationships (Wiley, London 1980).
Saltz, E.: Pretend play; a complex of variables influencing development. Annu. Meet. Am. Psychol. 1980.
Schlosberg, H.: The concept of play. Psychol. Rev. *54:* 229–231 (1947).
Spencer, W.: Principles of psychology; vol. 2 (Appleton, New York 1873).
Sutton-Smith, B.: Piaget, play and cognition revisited; in Overton, The relationship between social and cognitive development (Erlbaum, New York, in press 1982).
Wolf, D.; Gardner, H.: Style and sequence in early symbolic play; in Smith, Franklin, Early symbolization (Erlbaum, Hillsdale, N.J. 1979).

Contr. hum. Dev., vol. 6, pp. 4–14 (Karger, Basel 1982)

Early Play Theories Revisited: Contributions to Contemporary Research and Theory

Kenneth H. Rubin
University of Waterloo, Waterloo, Ont., Canada

In recent years, researchers have examined theoretically based hypotheses that play serves a causal role in the development of such widely diverse skills as role-taking, quantitative invariance, language acquisition, problem-solving, creativity and divergent thinking [*Rubin* et al., 1982, for a review of this research]. Indeed, the volume in which this chapter appears is testimony to the plethora of recently gathered data in which correlational and causal links have been established between different forms of play and laboratory assessments of the aforementioned variables.

Interestingly, an examination of the extant published studies concerning the correlates and consequences of play reveals a consistent citation pattern. Those who investigate the relations between play and role-taking, quantitative invariance, language development and other indices of symbolic representation typically refer to *Piaget* [1962] or *Vygotsky* [1967] as providing the major theoretical impetus for their work. Other researchers typically indicate that the feelings of comfort, relaxation, and security engendered within the play context promote the diversive object exploration necessary for the development of problem-solving and/or creativity. The theorists generally cited in this area include *Berlyne* [1969], *Birch* [1945], *Bruner* [1972], *Hutt* [1976], *Schiller* [1957] and *Sutton-Smith* [1976]. Although these citations are, for the most part, well-taken, they nevertheless fail to provide the reader with insights as to the origins or roots of the cited theories. In short, the 'classical' nineteenth and early twentieth century theories of play are generally slighted when present-day psychologists attempt to provide their readers with the names or works of theorists who sparked their own research interests.

The neglect of the early theories may oft-times be purposeful, that is, in an attempt to save precious journal space the author may choose to cite only the most recent relevant theories. On the other hand, it is conceivable that present-day students of children's play have been overreliant on secondary sources when accruing knowledge about the classical theories. Given that the general tenets of these theories have been widely criticized over the years [*Ellis*, 1973], purposeful citation omission can be well understood. However, it is important to note that a first-hand reading of the theories reveals that many of the significant research-stimulating insights attributed to the well-known contemporary theorists actually find their origins or roots in the classical works. Thus, the purpose of this chapter is simply to establish a sense of theoretical continuity in the heavily studied area of children's play.

The 'classical' theories of play include (a) the surplus energy; (b) the practice, and (c) the recapitulation theories of play [*Berlyne*, 1969; *Gilmore*, 1971]. In each theory, the proponents have attempted to explain the origins of play and its significance for development. For readers interested in more expansive, descriptive treatments, excellent reviews and critical comments concerning the classical theories may be found in *Ellis* [1973], *Levy* [1977], and *Millar* [1968]. A brief description of each theory is presented, in turn, below.

The Surplus Energy Theory of Play

The belief that play is essentially 'blowing off steam' dates back to Ancient Greek philosophy and the Aristotelian concept of catharsis. However, the first 'classical' treatment of the theory may be found in the writings of *Friedrich von Schiller*, an eighteenth century poet and philosopher who is far better known for his poem 'Ode to Joy' (upon which *Beethoven* based the last movement of his Ninth Symphony) than for his treatise on play. *Schiller's* interest in play emanated from his primary concern with aesthetic education. In his letters entitled *On the Aesthetic Education of Man*, *Schiller* [1954] defined play as 'the aimless expenditure of exuberant energy'. *Schiller's* major tenet was that people worked to satisfy their primary, appetitive needs. Play was viewed as the product of the superfluous energy left over once the primary needs were met. Children, because they were not responsible for their own survival, were considered to have a total energy 'surplus' which was depleted through play.

A number of contemporary issues concerning play were introduced in

Schiller's writings. For one, he noted that the purpose of play was to establish a sense of aesthetic appreciation in humankind. Play was considered to be the medium through which the player could transform and transcend reality thereby gaining new symbolic representations of the world. Given *Schiller's* views, contemporary play enthusiasts can readily identify a connection with the theoretical speculations of *Piaget* [1962], *Vygotsky* [1967] and *Singer* [1973] among others.

A second present-day issue found in *Schiller's* letters concerns the distinction he made between different types of play. He introduced the term 'Überfluss', or material superfluity, which purportedly resulted in physical play. As described by *Schiller*, this form of activity resembled *Bühler's* [1928] and *Piaget's* [1962] category of functional play. Aesthetic superfluity, on the other hand, culminated in aesthetic or dramatic/symbolic play [*Lieberman*, 1977], another category that appears in *Piaget's* [1962] *Play, Dreams and Imitation in Childhood.* Incidentally, it is noteworthy that the oft-cited Piagetian categories of play, which were elaborated by *Smilansky* [1968], i.e., functional, constructive, and dramatic play actually derive from *Bühler's* [1928] definitions of 'Funktionsspiele', 'Konstruktionsspiele', and 'Fiktionsspiele', respectively. Thus, the roots of present-day observational play coding schemes [*Lieberman*, 1977; *Rubin* et al., 1976a, b] can be traced, in part, back to the early nineteenth century letters of *Schiller*.

Spencer [1873], a nineteenth century British philosopher and psychologist, wrote that his thoughts about play evolved from reading the works of a German author whose name he could not remember. This common citation problem led *Groos* [1898] and other major early twentieth century contributors to the play literature [*Bowen and Mitchell*, 1924] to assume that the German author was none other than *Schiller*. In fact, a number of writers could have ignited the spark which led *Spencer* [1873] to write about play including *Fröbel* [1890] and *Jean Paul* [1892]. At any rate, following the publication of *Groos*' [1901] classic text, *The Play of Animals*, *Spencer* became accredited with the first psychological expression of the 'surplus energy' theory of play . . . a credit which, as the reader will note, was neither fair nor warranted.

Spencer's theory was drawn from his interest in what he believed to be a universal tendency for animals and humankind to be active. In his chapter on the development of the nervous system, *Spencer* [1873] wrote that with mental and physical activity, nerve cells are torn down. These cells were thought to gradually repair and rebuild themselves through quiescence. *Spencer* further believed that when the cells are replenished, there is a renewed readiness for the organism to act. Since revitalized cells are especially sensitive to stimulation, the result is an almost uncontrollable desire for action.

Spencer further postulated that the actions engaged in by the replenished organism would vary according to its status in the phylogenetic hierarchy. Thus, with increased status proportionally less time was spent 'absorbed in providing for immediate needs'. Given that less nervous energy was expended to maintain life among 'higher' than 'lower' animals, the former group had more energy to discharge on non-life-supporting endeavors. These latter activities, carried on without regard to ulterior benefit and spurred on by the replenished or revitalized nerves, were labelled 'play'.

It is interesting to note that in the few pages devoted to a discussion of play, *Spencer* [1873], himself, never used the term 'surplus energy'. Instead, he wrote that play is the superfluous and useless exercise of the nerve cells that have been quiescent. Thus, play as 'superfluous activity' belongs to *Spencer*. It would appear as if the notion of surplus energy rightfully belongs to *Schiller* and, accordingly, to *Groos* [1898], who popularized the theory in *Spencer's* name.

Groos [1898] was also responsible for suggesting that *Spencer* saw a strong tendency for the play of children to be imitative of the 'works' of adults. This, too, is a somewhat incorrect conception of *Spencer's* theory, which has persisted in the writings of play historians during this century. Actually, *Spencer* appears to have been an instinct theorist who saw play as being the unconscious product of such life-satisfying, inborn instincts as the desire for conquest and dominance. Thus, when there was little demand for the literal activities of the instinctively based behaviors in childhood, the young of the species produced nonliteral analogues, without necessarily having seen the literal behavior displayed by an adult. An example cited was the play fight or the rough-and-tumble play of young boys. Given that the different forms of play described by *Spencer* were supposedly accounted for by varying inborn instincts, the theory comes far closer to that of *Hall* [1920] than to that of *Schiller* – a point that will be highlighted in the discussion of recapitulation theory.

Perhaps *Spencer's* most interesting, but heretofore least known contribution to play theory was the distinction he made between different forms of the phenomenon. On a single, illuminating page in his *Principles of Psychology*, *Spencer* [1873] introduced (and went no further than an introduction) (a) the superfluous activity of the sensorimotor apparatus; (b) artistic-aesthetic play; (c) the higher coordinating powers of games, and (d) mimicry.

The first two forms of play strongly resemble *Bühler's* [1928] categories of 'Funktionsspiele' and 'Fiktionsspiele' and *Piaget's* [1962] categories of practice and symbolic play. The latter two forms of play appear analogous to *Piaget's* categories of games with rules and imitation. Thus, with *Spencer*, as with *Schiller* before him, we see the roots of *Piaget's* cognitively oriented play theory.

SUPPORT TOLMAN

Finally, a number of twentieth century psychologists have offered theoretical, if not experimental, support for the surplus energy theory. *Tolman* [1932], for example, suggested that once the primary needs for food, sex, contact, and rest were met, the organism would find itself in a physiologically homeostatic condition. However, if quiescence lasted for too long a period of time, the organism would find itself in a condition of having too much unspent energy. *Tolman* wrote that the secondary needs for play or aesthetic satisfaction, when pressed into action, could alleviate the negative condition of having surplus energy.

CRITS OF SURPLUS ENERGY

Over the years, proponents of the surplus energy theory have been criticized by theorists and researchers alike. At the most basic level, there does not appear to be any empirical support for the existence of a hydraulic-energy system functioning within the human species, *Beach* [1945]. And yet, *Berlyne's* [1960] provocative theory of arousal motivation rests squarely on the assumption that neural needs and their satisfaction are responsible for exploratory and play activities. In this regard, it is important to distinguish between *Schiller's* view of play as resulting from a surplus of energy and *Spencer's* notion that play is superfluous activity resulting from neural quiescence.

Other criticisms for the surplus energy theory abound. Reviews of these critical comments may be found in *Ellis* [1973], *Levy* [1977] and *Rubin* et al. [1982]. Since it is my intent to simply explore the historical extensions of the classical theories, I will not touch upon the critical comments offered in other sources herein.

The Practice (Preexercise) Theory of Play

The second classical theory that has bearing on contemporary play research was best articulated by *Groos* [1898, 1901]. To this self-acknowledged neo-Darwinian, play had to serve an adaptive purpose for it to have continued its existence over the years in various species. *Groos*, in fact, suggested that play was the very 'stuff' of childhood, and that the period of childhood (or immaturity) existed in order that the organism may play. Moreover, the length of this play period was postulated to vary in direct accord with the organism's place in the phylogenetic domain; the more complex the organism, the longer its period of immaturity. The longer periods of immaturity in more complex species were considered necessary to allow the practice of those instinctively based skills which were necessary for survival during adulthood. *Groos* thus presented the view that play existed to allow the practice of adaptive activities – a view in keeping with contemporary developmental theory [*Bruner*, 1972].

In outlining his position vis-à-vis the existence of play, *Groos* quickly dismissed the surplus energy theory described above. Play was considered adaptive and necessary for the survival of the species rather than an aimless discharge of surplus energy (the latter of which was *Groos*' interpretation of *Spencer's* writings). Play existed so that the young of the species could practice instinctively based behaviors. Obviously, for some animals instinctive behaviors arrived fully developed on first trial. As a result, there was no need for a period of play to exist for them. However, for other, more complex organisms, the life-sustaining instincts emerged in an undeveloped fashion during childhood. Play thus allowed the exercise, elaboration, and perfection of these behaviors before they became necessary for survival in adulthood.

Given the current revival of interest in the works of *Baldwin* [1906], it is noteworthy that this scholar wrote the preface for *Groos*' [1898] epic *The Play of Animals*. As in *Baldwin's* early formulation of the derivation of imitation, *Groos* suggested that play, too, emanated from a general instinctual impulse. Like *Baldwin's* theory of the function of imitation, *Groos* suggested that play served to elaborate other primitively, but more specifically developed instincts. Thus play, through the elaboration of undeveloped instinctual behaviors, allowed the emergence of intelligent, nonreflective behaviors in higher species. For *Groos*, a direct consequence of children's play was the development of intelligent behavior – again, a view shared by many contemporary psychologists and educators.

Having described *Groos*' viewpoint concerning the functions of play we now turn to his definition of the phenomenon. *Groos*, as did *Spencer*, considered children's play to be comprised of 'don't-have-to' activities. He suggested that while playing children were more interested in the processes than in the products of the behavior. The work of *White* [1959] and others concerned with effectance motivation thus finds its historical roots in these early writings.

Groos [1901] also developed a category system for examining the forms and functions of children's play. Experimental play, which included sensory and motor practice and practice of the higher mental powers (actually a 'games-with-rules' category), served the purpose of developing self-control. Socionomic play included fighting and chasing ('rough-and-tumble' play) and imitative, social and family games (dramatic play). This latter category was postulated to aid in the development of interpersonal skills, a hypothesis in keeping with contemporary views of the causal benefits of fantasy and dramatic play [*Rubin and Pepler*, 1980; *Singer*, 1973; *Smilansky*, 1968].

The Recapitulation Theory of Play

The third classical theory to be described herein derives from the writings of *Hall* [1920], who is generally acknowledged to be the 'father' of the North American child psychology movement. *Hall* believed that child development provided a means for detecting both between- and within-species evolution. With embryonic growth, humans were thought to retrace their evolutionary paths from protozoan to human. During childhood play, the history of humankind could be progressively recapitulated. Thus, for example, those childhood games which involved running, throwing, and club hitting (baseball) were viewed as modern extensions of earlier racial hunting activities.

To *Hall*, the function of play was cathartic in nature. It was suggested that during the early years of life, children 'played out' their racial instincts. Such displays of behavior were thought to weaken the instincts derived from earlier epochs thereby allowing the development of more complex forms of activity typical of modern civilizations.

It is interesting to note that *Hall* [1920] viewed *Groos*' [1901] notion that play was practice for adult relevant activities as 'very partial, superficial, and perverse' because it ignored the historical past. Yet, in some ways, the two theories are indirectly related to mid-twentieth century and present-day psychoanalytic views of play.

In *Groos*' case, the view that children's play allowed the practice and mastery of adult relevant behaviors may be linked to the speculation of *Freud* [1961] that play allowed the mastery of anxiety-producing events. To *Freud*, individuals were thought to master the traumatic events of childhood through the compulsive repetition of the behavioral and contextual components of these events. If children were not allowed to master these traumatizing events through their play, they were considered to be 'at risk'

the research of those who advance pretense activities for lower SES children in order to ameliorate or to prevent social and cognitive deficits [*Rubin* et al., in press; *Saltz and Brodie*, this volume, for reviews of this work].

In conclusion, my major goal in writing this chapter was simply to describe some of the historical roots of contemporary research and theory concerning children's play. If I have been partially successful in reaching my goal, then readers of this chapter should have a historical appreciation for those contemporary issues raised and resolved in the remaining chapters of this volume.

References

Axline, V.: Play therapy (Ballantyne, New York 1969).

Baldwin, J.M.: Social and ethical interpretations of mental development (Macmillan, New York 1906).

Bateson, G.: The message 'This is play'; in Schaffner, Group processes (Macy, New York 1956).

Beach, F.A.: Current concepts of play in animals. Am. Nat. *79:* 523–541 (1945).

Berlyne, D.: Conflict, arousal and curiosity (McGraw-Hill, New York 1960).

Berlyne, D.: Laughter, humor, and play; in Lindzey, Aronson, The handbook of social psychology; vol. 3 (Addison-Wesley, Reading, Mass. 1969).

Birch, H.G.: The relation of previous experience to insightful problem-solving. J. comp. Psychol. *38:* 267–283 (1945).

Bowen, W.P.; Mitchell, E.D.: The theory of organized play (Barnes, New York 1924).

Bruner, J.S.: The nature and uses of immaturity. Am. Psychol. *27:* 687–708 (1972).

Bühler, C.: Kindheit und Jugend (Hirzel, Leipzig 1928).

Dansky, J.L.: Make believe: a mediator of the relationship between play and associative fluency. Child Dev. *51:* 576–579 (1980).

Ellis, M.: Why people play (Prentice-Hall, Englewood Cliffs, N.J. 1973).

Fein, G.G.: A transformational analysis of pretending. Devl Psychol. *11:* 291–296 (1975).

Freud, S.: Beyond the pleasure principle (Norton, New York 1961).

Fröbel, F.: Autobiography (Bardeen, Syracuse 1890).

Garvey, C.: Play (Harvard University Press, Cambridge 1977).

Gilmore, J.B.: Play: a special behavior; in Herron, Sutton-Smith, Child's play (Wiley, New York 1971).

Griffing, P.: The relationship between socioeconomic status and sociodramatic play among black kindergarten children. Genet. Psychol. Monogr. *101:* 3–34 (1980).

Groos, K.: The play of animals (Appleton, New York 1898).

Groos, K.: The play of man (Appleton, New York 1901).

Gulick, L.: A philosophy of play (Scribners, New York 1898).

Hall, G.S.: Youth (Appleton, New York 1920).

Hutt, C.: Exploration and play in children; in Bruner, Jolly, Sylva, Play: its role in development and evolution (Penguin, Middlesex 1976).

Jean Paul: Levana (Beyer, Langensalza 1892).

Lee, J.P.: Play in education (Macmillan, New York 1915).

Levy, J.: Play behavior (Wiley, New York 1977).

Lieberman, J.N.: Playfulness: its relationship to imagination and creativity (Academic Press, New York 1977).

Millar, S.: The psychology of play (Penguin, Baltimore 1968).

Piaget, J.: Play, dreams and imitation in childhood (Norton, New York 1962).

Rosen, C.E.: The effects of sociodramatic play on problem-solving behavior among culturally disadvantaged children. Child Dev. *45:* 920–927 (1974).

Rubin, K.H.; Fein, G.G.; Vandenberg, B.: Play; in Hetherington, Handbook of child psychology: social development; 4th ed. (Wiley, New York, in press 1982).

Rubin, K.H.; Maioni, T.L.; Hornung, M.: Free play behaviors in middle and lower class preschoolers: Parten and Piaget revisited. Child Dev. *47:* 414–419 (1976a).

Rubin, K.H.; Pepler, D.J.: The relationship of child's play to social-cognitive development; in Foot, Chapman, Smith, Friendship and childhood relationships (Wiley, London 1980).

Rubin, K.H.; Watson, K.; Jambor, T.: Free play behaviors in preschool and kindergarten children. Child Dev. *47:* 414–419 (1976b).

Schiller, F.: On the aesthetic education of man (Yale University Press, New Haven 1954).

Schiller, P.H.: Innate motor action as a basis of learning; in Schiller, Instinctive behavior (International Universities Press, New York 1957).

Singer, J.L.: The child's world of make believe: experimental studies of imaginative play (Academic Press, New York 1973).

Smilansky, S.: The effects of sociodramatic play on disadvantaged preschool children (Wiley, New York 1968).

Smith, P.K.; Dodsworth, C.: Social class differences in the fantasy play of preschool children. J. genet. Psychol. *133:* 183–190 (1978).

Spencer, W.: Principles of psychology; vol. 2 (Appleton, New York 1873).

Sutton-Smith, B.: Current research and theory on play, games and sports, exercise and recreation (American Medical Association, Chicago 1976).

Sylva, K.; Bruner, J.; Genova, P.: The role of play in the problem-solving of children 3–5 years old; in Bruner, Jolly, Sylva, Play – its role in development and evolution (Penguin, New York 1976).

Tolman, E.C.: Purposive behavior in animals and men (Century, New York 1932).

Vygotsky, L.S.: Play and its role in the mental development of the child. Soviet Psychol. *12:* 62–76 (1967).

White, R.W.: Motivation reconsidered: the concept of competence. Psychol. Rev. *66:* 297–323 (1959).

Contr. hum. Dev., vol. 6, pp. 15–20 (Karger, Basel 1982)

Play: A Concept in Need of a Definition?

Brian Vandenberg

University of Missouri, St. Louis, Mo., USA

Fools, comedians and clowns are a culture's way of making fun of itself. People in these roles are allowed to poke fun at the traditional myths and symbols of a culture and are given this license because it is 'all in fun'. Despite the levity (or perhaps because of it), a culture's clowns are the source of important insights into that culture. In some ways, 'play' is a clown in the realm of psychological phenomena. It has eluded precise formulation, and at times seems to be playing hide-and-seek with us. We respond by either dismissing it as an unimportant prankster, or by trying harder to find it. But like the clown, its pranks also uncover basic assumptions. Play's playing with us raises fundamental questions about the nature of scientific definitions: Is ambiguity in defining a term, such as play, reason enough to reject it as a useful scientific concept? Are the problems of defining play significantly different from defining other psychological phenomena? What are the limits of definitional rigor? Are there alternative strategies that could be used to define play? Rather than try to identify or review those features of play which should be included in a definition of play [*Rubin* et al., 1982] I would like to pursue the deep message in our inability to corner play: to review these epistemological questions raised by that clever fool, play.

Question: Does the failure to develop an unambiguous definition of play (or any other phenomenon) mean that it must be dismissed as a viable scientific concept?

This question is a consequence of the epistemological doctrine of operationalism. One of the axioms of operationalism is that the ontological status of an entity is contingent on whether a reliable, operational definition can be established. Consequently, our failure to operationalize 'play' means that it must be banished from the halls of science. The practice of operationalizing a term has proved to be of great help to psychology, as it has provided a way of establishing a firm footing for research. Unfortunately, it sometimes has been considered as the *only* means of establishing the ontological status of an entity. Operationalism is not equivalent to science; it is only one way of approaching scientific questions, and there are fundamental difficulties which suggest that we be cautious in our use of operational principles. Let me briefly summarize several of these difficulties.

It is a common belief among many social scientists that operationalism is the modus operandi of the physical sciences. The history of science, however, reveals that operationalism has had a rather brief and unsuccessful tenure within the physical sciences. One of the first uses of operationalism was by a 19th century chemist named *Brody*. He used it to define chemical processes and entities. So, for example, a chemical reaction was defined by the operations that the chemist performed to produce the reactions. *Brody* was an important chemist in his day, but today he is hardly known. His operational system for defining chemical phenomena was replaced by a less operational (and more 'mentalistic') notion – the atom.

There is also a logical problem with operationalism. If something must be operationalized before it can be entertained as a viable scientific concept, then how is the principle of operationalism itself justified? In the end, we have to say that the reasons for adopting operationalism are arbitrary, or at least subjective. Thus, in attempting to eliminate subjectivity, we have only displaced it. The question then becomes: 'Which do we have more faith in – the principles of operationalism or the phenomena being operationalized?' In the case of play, this means that we can either conclude that the failure to derive a reliable, operational definition of play means that we must eliminate this concept from our scientific universe, or that the failure to include play in our scientific universe reflects a reductio ad absurdum of the principles used to determine scientific credibility. I must say that I am more conficent of the status of play as a real entity than I am of the doctrine of operationalism.

It is rather curious that we should hinge the ontological status of play (or any other phenomenon) on our ability to define it precisely. I am reminded of the story of the man who one night lost his keys, and asked a friend to help him try to find them. After spending time searching the area around the streetlight, the friend asked the man if he had been in the area they were searching when he lost his keys. The man replied that, no, he had not been in that area, but he was searching there because he could see better where the light was. Similarly, we can search for play under the streetlight of operationalism, but our failure to find it there does not preclude its existence.

Although it is uncomfortable, unfortunate and untidy that play has eluded a precise operational formulation (some might argue that this is its allure), it is certainly not unprecedented. The definition of light has proved to be a puzzle for physicists for centuries. Under some circumstances it acts as a wave, and under other conditions it acts as a particle. Which is it? How shall we define it? How can this logical contradiction be resolved? The failure to define light in an unambiguous way has not resulted in our dismissing light as a nonentity. Rather, it has led to a greater appreciation of the complexity, subtlety and magic of this phenomenon. Play, like light, is not easily corralled, and the difficulty in defining these terms is not an ipso facto reason for dismissing them as 'unscientific'.

Question: Are the problems of defining play significantly different than those encountered when trying to define other phenomena?

I think not, but our cultural attitudes toward play may influence our scientific judgments about play. *Berlyne* [1969] has pointed out that play is a term which refers to a large number of disoarate behaviors, and he suggests that this is sufficient reason to dispense with the term 'play' altogether. However, there are many other behaviors studied by psychologists that are equally broad, but which have not aroused the skepticism that play has. Take aggression, for example. There are many forms of aggression: physical aggression, verbal aggression, aggressive postures, aggressive or hostile humor, play fights, passive aggressive acts and hostile intentions are some that come to mind. It is probably impossible to provide an operational definition of aggression that could incorporate all of these behaviors, but few would conclude that we should refrain from using the term 'aggression'. Fewer still would conclude that our failure means that there is no such thing as aggression. A quick perusal of the evening paper tells us otherwise.

The same evening paper also contains the sports and the comics. Unfortunately, these sections are usually buried in the deep recesses of the paper, and their placement reflects how our culture values play as a frivolous diversion from the more important tasks in life. This attitude is also reflected in the research efforts of psychologists. Historically, aggression, intelligence and sex differences have been among the most highly researched topics in psychology. In comparison, play has been a much-neglected topic, not only in psychology, but in other social sciences as well [*Schwartzman*, 1978], and even in many of the current investigations there has been an implicit bias against play qua play.

For example, a recent American Psychological Association symposium was devoted to the question of whether play is a causal agent in the development of problem-solving skills. However, the question of whether play is a causal agent in development implies that play is the handmaiden for other, 'more important' aspects of development, such as problem-solving. The importance of play hinges on its relationship to this other, more culturally valued behavior. If play can be shown to influence this other variable, then by association it, too, must be important. The question being asked is whether play is really important, or whether it is just the useless and frivolous behavior it is commonly thought to be. By really important, we mean causal, and by causal, we mean does it have an effect on problem-solving and IQ-related behaviors whose importance is clearly recognized by the culture?

When was the last time a symposium was held on whether cognition is a causal agent in development? To frame the question this way seems odd. Cognition is not a causal agent in development – it is an important aspect *of* development. I suspect that we frame our questions about play in the way we do because we do not believe that play is an important aspect *of* development. I also think this attitude is responsible for our willingness to dispense with the term play as 'unscientific' when we might not be as quick to so judge other behaviors.

Question: Is an airtight definition possible in psychology?

The answer to this question depends, of course, on what is meant by 'airtight'. There are, however, some inherent limitations in our ability to precisely define a phenomenon. These limitations are exemplified in the attempts of mathematicians to define arithmetic in logical terms. For a number of centuries mathematicians struggled to develop axiomatically defined relationships that could be used to describe arithmetic. *Gödel* [*Crossley* et al., 1972], however, has demonstrated that such a system is impossible. *Gödel's* theorem, to paraphrase, states that no logical system which is powerful enough to contain arithmetic can demonstrate its own consistency, and that such a system allows for the generation of 'undecidable' proposition; that is, propositions whose truths cannot be determined within the system itself. Thus, even in the most perfect of systems, such as logic, uncertainty is inevitable.

A similar analogy can be found in physics. Under ordinary space-time-energy conditions, we can treat ourselves as investigators who are separate from the system we are measuring. This is the Newtonian universe, and is one that psychology frequently models itself after; the experimenter (the E) and the subjects (the Ss) are independent systems. The Newtonian world, however, breaks down under more unusual space-time-energy circumstances (which, from the universe's perspective, are more usual); we can no longer be treated as separate from the physical system we are examining, and we must consider *Heisenberg's* uncertainty principle, which quantifies the uncertainty that is generated when a physical system (the E) measures an aspect of itself (a particle).

In both logic and physics, uncertainty is a necessary consequence of a system attempting to measure or comment on itself. If we compare psychology to logic and physics, we have an even more complex set of problems. Here we have a system (E) measuring 'itself' (other humans, or Ss), and the part being measured is capable of being aware of being measured, and can alter its behavior accordingly. It is at least a dual level of self-reflection that should multiply the uncertainty enormously. Thus, there is uncertainty built into the self-referent definitional system of psychology – by definition. This is not really a new idea. *William James* as well as *Plato* have pointed out the problems and limitations of self-reflection, but *Gödel* and *Heisenberg* provide us with formalized proofs of the limits of self-reflective systems.

This is not, of course, an argument for abandoning our efforts to think precisely about the terms we use. The aspiration for a precise definition of play is an admirable impulse which will lead to further refinements in our conceptualization of the term. However, the belief that airtight definitions are ultimately possible may lead us to be impatient with imprecise definitions, and cause us to throw the playful baby out with the bathwater.

Question: Are there alternative ways of thinking about definitions?

Instead of trying to tie definitions to the concrete, we could try to move toward more formal, idealized conceptualizations which are independent of particular concrete manifestations of the definition. Although this sounds like *Plato*, it actually is a common strategy in science. For instance, *Newton's* second law states: $F = ma$. This fundamental law, until very recently, could never be directly demonstrated. It is an idealized relationship that is correct only in perfect vacuums (i.e., in an idealized system), and had to be altered to consider the perturbation effects of things like friction in the less idealized systems here on earth.

Perhaps we could consider the abstract, generalized definitions of play as the expression of the idealized form of play, whose particular manifestation is contingent upon cultural, contextual, developmental and interpersonal perturbating factors. The form that play takes varies as a function of these and other factors, and what is needed are efforts aimed at linking the abstract definition with its concrete manifestations, and an analysis of how the perturbating factors influence the specific form of play.

Matthews and Matthews [this volume] propose a novel way of using videotapes to define prototypical play behaviors which are used as standards for assessing whether other behaviors are to be considered 'play'. Their method serves as a useful alternative to the usual verbal, written methods of definition, and offers promise for bridging the gap between the abstract definition of play and its various behavioral manifestations.

In sum, the failure to define play is not a fatal flaw, and is as much a comment on our epistemological assumptions and methodologies as it is a comment on play. This realization should force us to be clear about what we expect from a definition, to explore new methodologies for defining play, and to value play as much as other, 'more important' psychological phenomena.

References

Berlyne, D.E.: Laughter, humor and play; in Lindzey, Aronson, The handbook of social psychology; vol. 3 (Addison-Wesley, Reading, Mass. 1969).

Crossley, S.N.; Ash, C.J.; Brickhill, C.J.; Stillwell, J.C.; Williams, N.H.: What is mathematical logic? (Oxford University Press, London 1972).

Rubin, K.; Fein, G.G.; Vandenberg, B.: Play; in Hetherington, Handbook of child psychology: social development (Wiley, New York, in press 1982).

Schwartzman, H.B.: Transformations: the anthropology of children's play (Plenum, New York 1978).

Contr. hum. Dev., vol. 6, pp. 21–29 (Karger, Basel 1982)

Eliminating Operational Definitions: A Paradigm Case Approach to the Study of Fantasy Play

Wendy Schempp Matthews[a], *Robert J. Matthews*[b]

[a] UMD-Rutgers Medical School, Piscataway, N.J., and
[b] Rutgers University, New Brunswick, N.J., USA

Escapades into outer space, showdowns in the old saloon, conversations with a teddy bear are all instances of children's behavior which we would identify as examples of fantasy play. Each has an 'as-if' quality which, though elusive, cues us to the fact that the behavior represents fantasy. The children behave as if they were astronauts preparing their craft for touchdown; they act as if they had the fastest guns in the West. They conspire with the teddy bear as if they were in the company of a fellow master spy. And upon viewing behavior of this kind, we can agree in each case that 'that is a case of fantasy if anything is!' So why require an operational definition?

The methodological requirement that theoretical terms such as 'play' be operationally defined grows out of the behaviorism that for several decades dominated experimental psychology. Operational definitions are thought to be necessary if psychologists are 'to be rid of the hazy ambiguities which result in ceaseless argument and dissension' [*Stevens*, 1935a]. Operational definitions are intended to secure interresearcher agreement on terminology by associating with each term a concrete experimental operation or measurement. However, recent empirical research, for example in cognitive psychology, impugns the methodological rationale for operational definition; high interresearcher agreement should be obtainable without the use of operational definitions. Far from having the intended salutary effect on research methodology, operational definitions have often proved pernicious, especially in research directed towards the study of spontaneous behavior in naturalistic settings. In research on children's spontaneously occurring fantasy play, in lieu of operationism we employed a 'paradigm case approach' consonant with the results of recent research in cognitive psychology and elsewhere.

Operational Definitions

The requirement that theoretical terms be operationally defined arose during the 1930s in response to persistent doubts as to the scientific respectability of psychology. Under the influence of operationism and logical positivism, psychologists such as *Skinner*, *Spence*, *Stevens*, and *Tolman* attributed the unsatisfactory state of psychology to its lack of rigor in the formulation of fundamental concepts [*Stevens*, 1935b]. The cure, they believed, lay in the use of operational definitions which would provide precise, unambiguous definitions of theoretical terms. The definitions would require a restricted observational vocabulary that mentioned only concrete operations of a sort that could be easily replicated by other researchers. The empirical content of psychological theories formulated in an operationally defined theoretical vocabulary would presumably be both guaranteed and unambiguous.

The empirical impoverishment of preoperational psychological theorizing did indeed require attention; however, the operationalistic cure was unsatisfactory. As philosophers and psychologists eventually realized [*Ginsberg*, 1955; *Hempel*, 1965], the operationalistic demand for the explicit definition of theoretical terms restricted to an observational vocabulary was unsatisfiable. Even the theoretical terms of physics, chemistry, and biology could not be defined in this way. In attempting to formulate an adequate criterion for empirical significance, philosophers of science have found it necessary to retrench repeatedly, to the point that there now remains little of the original positivist/operationalistic requirement of explicit definability. All that remains is the modest requirement that theories be testable, i.e., that they have observational consequences that are subject to empirical test.

In highly theoretical domains of psychology, notably cognitive psychology, one now finds little mention of operational definitions. Some researchers speak of 'operationalizing a hypothesis', but this comes to nothing more than deriving a testable prediction from the hypothesis. Talk of operational definition remains widespread, however, in those domains that are concerned primarily with descriptive studies of behavior. As *Vandenberg* [this volume] points out, operational definitions are assumed to be methodologically necessary if the researcher is to identify the phenomenon under study clearly and unambiguously. Thus, in research directed towards the study of spontaneous behavior (e.g., play, empathy, aggression, coyness, etc.), discussions of research methodology will often begin with what are termed operational definitions of the phenomena under study. Strictly speaking, the proffered definitions are rarely operational, since they are couched in much less restrictive observational vocabulary than that countenanced by operationists. Nevertheless, the use to which these definitions are put is operationalistic in spirit: They stipulate what is to count as an instance of the behavior under study, and the stipulation is formulated in a basically observational vocabulary. The research findings are to be interpreted as descriptive of behavior that satisfies the stipulative definition.

The rationale for undertaking research directed towards the study of spontaneous behavior is to achieve a better understanding of the particular behavior under study. Usually this is taken to involve the provision of both a principled description of the behavior itself (e.g., its frequency, structure, content, etc.) as well as of its etiology. Furthermore, one expects the resulting description to provide a principled way of deciding precisely which behaviors are instances of the behavior under study (much as physical chemists used the results of their research on gold to determine whether everything that had heretofore been taken to be gold was in fact gold). The methodological difficulty with operational definitions is that they frustrate these research aims: By beginning with a definition of the behavior under study they effectively preclude the possibility of discovering that the behavior is more appropriately characterized in a manner different from the stipulated definition. After all, unless the operational definition was validated against pretheoretical judgments as to which behaviors were instances of the behavior under study, there is no reason to take the research findings to characterize anything except that behavior which satisfies the operational definition. Thus, to the extent that research is necessary to improve our identification and understanding of the behavior under study, research under the operationalistic paradigm will be unilluminating. Much recent research on spontaneous behavior, especially that conducted in a naturalistic setting, suffers from the methodological difficulty described: The operational definitions are wide of their mark; and as a result, the research designs based on these definitions preclude use of the research findings to revise the definitions.

The Paradigm Case Approach

The notion that operational definitions are necessary in order to secure high interresearcher agreement on the applicability of theoretical terms rests on specific *empirical* assumptions as to the acquisition, structure, and use of concepts. In particular, concepts (including theoretical concepts) were assumed to be unstructured feature lists that provided necessary and sufficient conditions for the application of the correlative terms. Recognition of instances falling under a concept was assumed to involve recognizing that the instances satisfied all (or most) of the defining conditions. High interresearcher agreement was assumed to require defining conditions the satisfaction of which could readily be ascertained by publicly replicable observations.

Recent research [*Posner* et al., 1967; *Posner and Keele*, 1968; *Rosch*, 1973, 1978; *Rosch and Mervis*, 1975] suggests strongly that these assumptions are not well-founded, at least not for many concepts of natural language. Such 'natural' concepts are not unstructured feature lists, nor are their boundaries well-defined. Rather, membership in the extension of the concept is defined in terms of similarity to prototypical instances of the concept. Recognition seemingly involves an appeal to a similarity metric defined on the prototypes: Something is recognized as an instance of the concept just in case it is sufficiently (and relevantly) similar to prototypical instances of that concept. Although the structure of only a limited number of natural concepts, chiefly categorical concepts, has thus far been investigated, it seems very likely that most natural language concepts will be found to have a similar structure, since these concepts are invariably acquired on the basis of exposure to a limited number of instances of the concept. If so, then the high intersubjective agreement that *Rosch* and others have noted on prototype recognition tasks can be expected to hold for many natural concepts. This suggests that if researchers focus on prototypical instances of a particular type of behavior, there should be high interresearcher agreement of just the sort that operational definitions were intended to secure.

Fantasy Play: An Application of the Approach

Research designs of reported studies of fantasy play typically incorporate an operational definition which purportedly delimits the domain of the study. Careful examination of the proposed definitions invariably reveals that the class of behaviors satisfying the definition is not coextensive with what would be pretheoretically recognized as the class of fantasy play behaviors. In some cases the operationally defined class of behaviors proves to be a proper subclass of fantasy play; in other cases, the operationally defined class contains fantasy as a proper subclass. But most commonly the operationally defined class of behaviors intersects the class of fantasy play behaviors: Clear cases of nonfantasy play are subsumed by the operational definition, while clear cases of fantasy play fail to be subsumed by the definition. *Markey's* [1935, p. 10] often cited definition of fantasy play provides a clear example of an overly broad definition. If, as she proposes, fantasy play behaviors are 'instances in which the child, through his language or overt behavior, dealt with objects, materials, activities, and situations as though they had properties or attributes other than those which they apparently or actually seemed to possess', then, for example, the child's use of a block as a hammer with which to pound a rubber tricycle handle more securely onto the handle bars should be construed for research purposes as an instance of fantasy play. Also included would be the behavior of a child who for one reason or another incorrectly attributes to some object, material, activity, or situation, properties that it does not possess. Surely every unintentional misinterpretation of a situation or object should not be counted an instance of fantasy!

Given the recognized failure of proposed operational definitions to define a class of behaviors coextensive with the class of fantasy play behaviors, operational definitions have become little more than methodological window dressing. Some researchers eschew them altogether. *Klinger* [1971], for example, notes that 'nearly everyone understands what is meant by "play", and investigators are even able substantially to agree in identifying particular instances'. 'But', he laments, 'positive definitions of play are quite divergent, often bound up in theoretical positions, and highly ambiguous at their boundaries' [pp. 17, 18]. Abandoning any effort to define play, *Klinger* attempts instead to define what play is *not:* 'play is defined here as behavior other than . . .' [p. 20]. In lieu of an operational definition, *Gilmore* [1966] substitutes a single behavioral example (e.g., that of a child putting a blanket 'to sleep'), which he assumes will indicate satisfactorily the class of behaviors under study.

The first author was faced with a similar dilemma in research on fantasy in the spontaneous play of young children. While recognizing the inadequacy of operational definitions, she nonetheless recognized the need to provide an intersubjectively reliable characterization of the domain of behaviors being studied. A paradigm case approach was adopted in lieu of an operational definition. *Black* [1976] explains the notion of a paradigm case as follows: 'By a "paradigm case" of the application of a given word, *W*, I mean some actual or possible thing, produced or merely described, of which it is correct to say, "that is a case of *W* if anything is!" ' A paradigm case, *Black* [1976] goes to say, is '(i) clear or central (as opposed to borderline); (ii) plain or obvious (as opposed to only inferentially a case of *W*; (iii) uncontroversial (not problematic); (iv) exemplary or standard – a case by reference to which a question whether something else is a case of *W* might properly be decided.'

Paradigm cases of fantasy play are behavioral instances which everyone, regardless of his or her theoretical or empirical bent, should agree are cases of fantasy. By restricting consideration to paradigm cases of fantasy play, the first author hypothesized that she would maintain high intersubjective agreement of just the sort envisioned by the requirement for operational definitions. Moreover, this agreement would be secured without the risk of experimental bias posed by the a priori construction of a definition of the behavior under study. To test the reliability of the paradigm case approach, 4 naive observers (i.e., individuals out of the field of psychology, with little or no experience with children) served to test the reliability of the paradigm case approach to the study of fantasy in the play of young children. The observers included 2 males (a bookstore clerk and a medical student) and 2 females (a librarian and a science student). By a 'paradigm case' of fantasy play was meant, to paraphrase *Black* [1976], some actual or possible instance of fantasy play, produced or merely described, of which it is correct to say, 'That is a case of *fantasy play* if anything is!'

The spontaneous interactions of eight same-sex pairs of 4-year-old children in three 1-hour play sessions in the naturalistic setting of a laboratory/playroom were observed and recorded on videotape. From the dyadic interactions, 90 paradigm cases of fantasy play were identified. These cases which, it is contended here, all observers would agree to be instances of fantasy play, thus represent the data corpus for related studies of fantasy play.

To prove the contention that the 90 cases of fantasy play were indeed instances of fantasy play upon which all would agree (without having to rely upon an operational definition), the following procedure was employed: Each of the 4 observers was asked to view eight 15-min segments of the videotapes of the children's interaction. The segments were randomly selected from the 24 h of recorded interaction, with the stipulation that each of the eight pairs of children, each of the play sessions (I, II, III), and each half of the sessions (early, late) be equally represented. The observer was provided with a brief description of the paradigm case approach, namely that it is a procedure for the identification of fantasy according to which it would be correct to say of an instance of fantasy play, 'That is a case of fantasy play if anything is!' The observer was then instructed in the use of a videotape playback unit and monitor and was left alone in the room with the instruc-

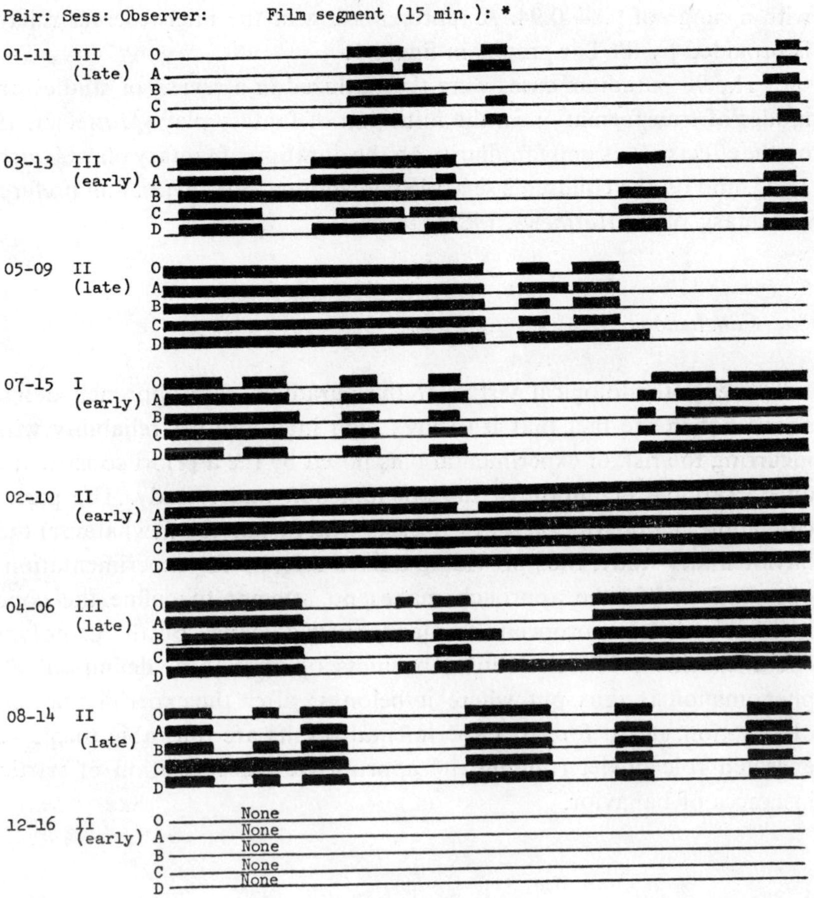

Fig. 1. Interobserver agreement regarding judgments of behavior as fantasy. The shaded areas represent time judged to be spent in fantasy.

tions to simply write a description when they thought the behavior they were viewing was fantasy play and to stop writing when they considered the fantasy play to have come to an end.

For purposes of analysis each of the eight 15-min film segments was divided into 30 half-minute units, for a total of 240 units which were judged by each of 5 observers (the 4 naive observers and the experimenter) to be either fantasy or nonfantasy. A phi coefficient was then computed to compare each observer with all the others. The average coefficient was 0.89

with a range of 0.84–0.94. A representation of the interobserver reliability is provided by the bar graphs in figure 1.

The 90 paradigm cases were then utilized in a review of studies on the modes of transformation in the initiation of fantasy play [*Matthews*, 1977], on the effects of sex and familiarity on the duration of fantasy play [*Matthews*, 1978], and on the children's sex-role perceptions, portrayals, and preferences in fantasy play [*Matthews*, 1981].

Conclusion

The methodological virtue of the paradigm case approach described above lies in the fact that it secures high interobserver reliability without incurring the risk of experimental bias posed by the a priori construction of an operational definition of the phenomenon under study. The paradigm case approach provides a set of prototypical instances of (whatever) the behavior under study, thus providing a fixed referent for experimentation and observation, but the approach makes no attempt to define the concept, inasmuch as the appropriate similarity metric defined on the prototypes is left unspecified. The theoretical business of offering a 'definition' of the phenomenon is thus put where it belongs: after the experimentation and observation, not before it. Experimental results are thus able to play their expected role of determining the appropriate categorization of particular instances of bahavior.

References

Black, M.· Paradigm cases and evaluative words; in Black, Critiques and caveats (Cornell University Press, Ithaca, N.Y. 1976).

Gilmore, J.B.: Play: a special behavior; in Haber, Current research in motivation, pp. 277–298 (Holt, Rinehart & Winston, London 1966).

Ginsberg, A.: Operational definitions and theories. J. gen. Psychol. *52:* 223–245 (1955).

Hempel, C.G.: Aspects of scientific explanation (Free Press, New York 1965).

Klinger, E.: Structure and functions of fantasy (Wiley-Interscience, New York 1971).

Markey, F.V.: Imaginative behavior of preschool children. Monogr. Soc. Res. Child Dev. *18:* 1–139 (1935).

Matthews, W.S.: Modes of transformation in the initiation of fantasy play. Devl Psychol. *13:* 212–216 (1977).

Matthews, W.S.: Sex and familiarity effects upon the proportion of time young children spend in spontaneous fantasy play. J. genet. Psychol. *133:* 9–12 (1978).

Matthews, W.S.: Sex-role perceptions, portrayal and preference in the fantasy play of young children. Sex Roles *7:* 979–987 (1981).

Posner, M.I.; Goldsmith, R.; Welton, K.E., Jr.: Perceived distance and the classification of distorted patterns. J. exp. Psychol. *73:* 23–28 (1967).

Posner, M.I.; Keele, S.W.: On the genesis of abstract ideas. J. exp. Psychol. *77:* 335–363 (1968).

Rosch, E.: On the internal structure of perceptual and semantic categories; in Moore, Cognitive development and the acquisition of language (Academic Press, New York 1973).

Rosch, E.: Principles of categorization; in Rosch, Lloyd, Cognition and categorization (New York 1978).

Rosch, E.; Mervis, C.B.: Family resemblances: studies in the internal structure of categories. Cognitive Psychol. *7:* 573–605 (1975).

Stevens, S.S.: The operational definition of psychological concepts. Psychol. Rev. *42:* 517–558 (1935a).

Stevens, S.S.: The operational basis of psychology. Am. J. Psychol. *47:* 323–330 (1935b).

Contr. hum. Dev., vol. 6, pp. 30–45 (Karger, Basel 1982)

Combinatorial Competency in Symbolic Play and Language

Lorraine McCune-Nicolich, Carol Bruskin[1]
Rutgers University, New Brunswick, N.J., USA

During the second year of life children make several transitions in mental development as they proceed from primarily sensorimotor to more representational or symbolic modes of functioning [*McCall* et al., 1977]. During this time children begin to use single-word speech, followed by simple verbal combinations. Previously [*McNeill*, 1970], it was generally assumed that such developments in language were entirely independent of transitions in other areas, and resulted from the unfolding of specific language-learning abilities.

However, recent theoretical and empirical work suggests that the underlying capacity to symbolize is influential in language development as well as in a variety of related areas. One such domain which appears to share cognitive components and task factors with language is the development of symbolic play. Thus the theories of development by *Piaget* [1962] and *Werner and Kaplan* [1963], which assume that underlying changes in cognitive structure lead to cross-domain effects on behavior, as well as those emphasizing more limited structural effects such as *Fischer* [1980] and *Bates* et al. [1977] would predict that a strong relationship should exist between domains such as language and symbolic play.

Correspondences between symbolic play and language have been proposed on theoretical grounds by *McCune-Nicolich* [1981], *Piaget* [1962] and *Werner and Kaplan* [1963]. In symbolic play, the child uses gestures, sounds and objects to represent or 'symbolize' other events and objects. In language, vocal-articulatory behaviors are used to represent and refer to objects and

[1] Helpful comments from *M. Braine*, *L. Fenson*, *D. Ramsay*, and *J. Raph* on an earlier draft are gratefully acknowledged.

events. Language and play also serve several joint functions in the second year of life. First, both involve the communicative function of sharing objects with others [*Dunn and Wooding*, 1977; *Werner and Kaplan*, 1963]. Second, children use both play and language to 'try out' various representational equivalences, and thereby learn the range of acceptable symbolic transformations. In the following paragraphs we will (1) describe the early development of symbolic play; (2) review recent research concerning relationships between symbolic play and language, and (3) propose hypotheses concerning specific underlying transitions in symbolic ability which may account for analogous developments in symbolic play and language. A study will then be reported which evaluates two of the proposed transitions.

Sequence of Developments in Symbolic Play

Following the course originally described by *Piaget* [1962], *Nicolich* [1977] has demonstrated an ordinal sequence of five levels in symbolic play: (1) presymbolic gestures showing understanding of the use of common objects; (2) onset of initial pretending related to the self; (3) extension of pretending to include behaviors observed in others, and the use of dolls as participants in play; (4) onset of combinatorial abilities in pretend, such that several participants (e.g., self, doll) are involved with a single action scheme or several actions are played in sequence, and (5) hierarchically organized play involving evidence that the external behavior observed was guided by a prior mental intention or transformation. The earliest of these behaviors is observed between 8 and 12 months of age, and the sequence of developments is ordinarily completed by 30 months of age. Evidence for the generality of this sequence from a large body of research was presented by *McCune-Nicolich* [1981]. In a recent paper *Belsky and Most* [1981] reported the scalability of a similar sequence of play behaviors.

Sequence of Developments in Language

Initial language development also occurs during the second and third years of life and begins with single words. Research concerning word combinations of children with a mean length of utterance (MLU) close to 2.0 [*Bloom*, 1970; *Bloom* et al., 1975; *Braine*, 1976; *Brown*, 1973] has demonstrated impressively consistent findings concerning the relationship of child semantic-syntactic development to the adult system. However, considerable controversy surrounds the nature of children's earliest verbal combinations, comprising the MLU range of 1.1–1.5 where little research evidence is available. It is unclear, for example, whether early combinations are rote-learned or based on some primitive semantic-syntactic system [*Bloom and Lahey*, 1978; *Crystal*, 1978; *Howe*, 1976]. Similarly, are 'true' combinations preceded by such transitional phenomena as 'successive single words' [*Bloom*, 1973; *Branigan*, 1979] and/or word repetition and the prefixing of phonological units to single words [*Dore*, 1975]? The broader perspective of cognitive development suggests that both play and language during this period reflect a system in transition from sensorimotor to symbolic functioning [*Edwards*, 1974].

Research Relating Symbolic Play and Language

A number of studies have supported strong correlations between symbolic play and language during the early stages of language acquisition by both normal and abnormal children. *Lowe and Costello* [1976] reported partial correlations (age statistically removed) of approximately 0.30 between symbolic play and two language scores, MLU and Reynell language score [*Reynell and Huntley*, 1971]. *Bates* et al. [1975] reported the co-occurrence of initial language and symbolic play in 2 subjects studied longitudinally. *Bates* et al. [1979] found that, between 9 and 13 months, symbolic play measures were the strongest predictors of gesture and language ability. *Fein* [1978] reported multivariate results demonstrating that symbolic play was closely associated with language production and comprehension, while other types of play were not. *Largo and Howard* [1979] reported positive correlations between pretend play and receptive language, while *Rosenblatt* [1977] found that children who learned language early engaged in more representational play than others. In addition, studies of autistic children [*Sigman and Ungerer*, 1980] and retarded children [*Jeffree and McConkey*, 1976; *Kahn*, 1975] found positive correlations between symbolic play and language measures, and recently a single study [*Steckol and Leonard*, in press] reported improvement in communicative competence following training in symbolic play.

The Hypothesis of Shared Structure

The thesis of the present paper is that the correlational evidence described above reflects several changes in underlying mental structure which influence specific language and play skills. *McCune-Nicolich* [1981] predicted that onset of single words in language would occur close in time to the initial single pretend behaviors comprising level 2 in symbolic play and that significant vocabulary growth would occur following the expansion of the symbolic capacity evident in level-3 play.

Two correspondences were also proposed between levels of symbolic play and development of multiword language. At level-4 play, when symbolic combinations are first observed, onset of simple verbal combinations is proposed. Such verbal combinations would involve learned routines and two-word sequences in which each word bears its own direct relationship to the nonlinguistic context, rather than reflecting knowledge of linguistic rules. According to *Werner and Kaplan* [1963], such early language constructions are based on a cognitive transition allowing several aspects of context to be (1) differentiated; (2) considered simultaneously, and (3) referenced sequentially with separate words. Thus, at their onset, combinations in both domains are proposed as linear and context-dependent. In play the child recreates sequences of behavior previously observed, or strings together actions involving a given object and several available 'actors'. In language, combinations are formed either on the basis of *linguistic* context (that is words occurring in sequence are learned as routines by the child) or the child simply mentions several aspects of the *nonlinguistic* context in sequence.

Later combinations, characteristic of level-5 play, are proposed as hierarchical, in the sense that a prior mental act guides the construction of a sequence of behaviors. In play, such prior acts involve an intention to carry out a symbolic behavior as indicated by announcement, search, or preparation. Children capable of hierarchically structuring symbolic play behaviors should also be capable of generating simple linguistic rules. Thus, in language, the 'prior act' is a linguistic rule of order inferred to exist on the basis of the distributional properties of the child's language.

Concerning the nature of such early rules, *Maratsos and Chalkley* [1980] proposed that children's first grammatical rule systems may derive from learning what specific words occur frequently in a fixed order. Later more abstract grammatical rules would be inferred from this type of word combination analysis. Such a theory is both compatible with the two-step sequence of development for early language combinations proposed in this paper and provides continuity between the single-word period and later grammar. Initial combinations (corresponding to level-4 play) would be either rote-learned, context-dependent, or both. Following this period, and corresponding to level-5 play, increased distancing of symbol from context would allow the generation of simple distributional rules [*Braine*, 1976] which form the basis for acquisition of the more complex and abstract linguistic rules observed in older children.

The research to be reported here tests for parallel transitions in the development of combinations in play and language. A number of qualitative comparisons of language occurring at level-4 versus level-5 play were made to assess the broader effects of more advanced symbolic capacity on language performance.

Method

Subjects were 5 girls ranging in age from 14 to 18 months at the time the study began. Samples of language and play 30 min long were videotaped monthly in the home from early in the single word period until multiword utterances comprised at least 50% of the child's verbalizations (table I). The method devised by *Bloom* [1970] was used to transcribe the mother and child language with accompanying contextual information. These transcripts were then judged according to the play analysis system and assigned one of five symbolic maturity levels.

Symbolic Play Assessment

Symbolic play was assessed using an observation instrument designed by *Nicolich* [1977], which is described in detail in a manual available from *McCune-Nicolich* [1981]. This approach is based on stages of symbolic play described by *Piaget* [1962]. When used with videotaped samples of free play behavior with a standard set of toys, this instrument yielded 0.85 interrater reliability for distinguishing the levels of symbolic play.

The behavior analyzed in this system begins with presymbolic gestures indicating an understanding of the realistic use of conventional objects such as comb, cup, spoon (level 1). All subsequent levels involve pretending. Children first pretend at single elements of their own activity (eating, sleeping, grooming; level 2). Next they re-create actions they have seen others perform, such as reading or feeding a baby (level 3). At this level dolls and animals are treated as participants in play. These behaviors are organized into sequences at level 4. At level 5 the new skill of planning pretend activities before executing them emerges. Subjects were assigned a symbolic level based on their most advanced spontaneous performance in the session. A more detailed report of the play results is available in *Nicolich* [1977].

Utterance Length

Utterance length in English words was determined by a coder who was naive concerning the play analysis. 'Allgone' and 'whatsat' were treated as single units, as is common in the language literature. With these exceptions, all utterances where two or more words shared a single intonation pattern, with terminal contour only on the final word, were considered 'combinations' for the purposes of this study.

Identifying Positional Patterns of Combination

All two-word utterances were analyzed according to procedures described by *Braine* [1976], with one modification. He analyzed the order of semantic constituents (such as 'actor-action') in two-word utterances, while the present analysis was applied to word order. Utterances longer than two words were reviewed to ascertain the effect of patterns discerned at the two-word level, and for the purpose of noting other apparent regularities.

A pattern is defined as 'positional' on statistical grounds if one order of the elements is significantly more frequent than the other possible order. Based on the binomial probability that each order is equally likely, a minimum of 6 utterances in the same order (with 0 in reverse order) is needed to demonstrate a pattern using a two-tailed test (at the 0.05 level of significance). If a given order is predicted, a one-tailed test yields significance at the 0.05 level with only a 5–0 distribution of order. If some utterances are in reverse order, a larger number of 'correctly ordered' utterances is required to demonstrate a significant pattern.

Results

The influence of underlying changes in symbolic ability on both play and language was supported by two types of findings. First, the onset of combinations in the two domains occurred close in time. Second, both qualitative and quantitative changes in language were associated with the attainment of level-5 play.

Onset of Combinatorial Ability in Symbolic Play and Language

Subjects in the present study consistently produced their first observed instance of verbal combination either at the same session as their first play combination or at a session following earlier demonstration of the ability to combine pretend play acts, a result significant at the 0.05 level by Fischer's exact test. 4 subjects showed neither ability at the beginning of the study. Janis and Meri produced their first language combinations in the session where they attained level-4 play. Mira and Shanti respectively showed a 1- and 2-month delay between attainment of level-4 play and use of verbal combinations. The fifth subject, Tracy, exhibited one or two combinations in both play and language at the initial observation session (table I).

Comparison of Language Samples at Levels 4 and 5

Utterance Length. MLU remained close to 1.1 during level-4 sessions, but rose dramatically (to 1.5 for Janis, Meri and Shanti; 1.3 for Tracy) within 2 months of entry into level-5 play. Mira demonstrated a spurt to MLU 1.6 four sessions after entering level-5 play (table I).

Utterance Frequency. The number of utterances for each child increased by at least 100% within one session of attaining level-5 play. Similarly the number of multiword types (different multiword utterances) increased by 200% in the session at which level-5 play was first observed. Janis and Tracy

Table I. Overview of the language samples

Age of child months	Level	Session	MLU	Total utterances	Total single-word types	Total multi-word types
Janis						
15.3		1	1.0	23	11	0
16.3		2	1.0	52	7	0
18	4	3	1.14	78	21	8
18.2		4	1.13	88	35	7
19.2		5	1.14	92	27	5
20.2		6	1.19	93	37	5
21.2	5	7	1.47	424	86	103
23		8	1.89	317	63	111
Meri						
15		1	1.00	33	13	0
16	4	2	1.02	91	25	1
16.3		3	1.02	120	36	1
17.3		4	1.07	83	32	5
18.2		5	1.03	171	71	3
19.3	5	6	1.17	296	70	29
21		7	1.54	372	74	97
Mira						
15		1	1.0	10	4	0
16.1	4	2	1.0	71	26	0
17.1		3	1.05	146	42	4
18	5	4	1.07	417	44	13
19		5	1.03	149	30	3
20.1		6	1.15	310	62	30
21.1		7	1.62	384	55	104
22.1		8	1.80	309	46	120
Shanti						
14.1		1	1.0	78	10	0
15.1	4	2	1.0	46	11	0
16.1		3	1.0	122	32	0
17.2		4	1.0	103	27	1
18.1		5	1.06	114	36	4
19		6	1.0	108	33	0
20		7	1.09	333	63	18

Table I. (continued)

Age of child months	Level	Session	MLU	Total utterances	Total single-word types	Total multi-word types
21	5	8	1.49	390	71	95
22		9	1.72	439	65	109
23		10	1.74	460	69	120
24		11	1.84	384	75	134
Tracy						
19		1	1.06	35	15	2
20		2	1.02	41	12	1
21.2		3	1.03	114	24	2
22.2		4	1.02	124	34	2
23.2	4	5	1.04	74	28	3
24.2		6	1.11	89	30	7
25		7	1.14	50	23	5
26	5	8	1.19	301	64	36
26.3		9	1.31	218	57	38
27.3		10	1.31	318	65	67

also produced more than twice as many single words in their first level-5 session than they had previously produced (table I).

It can be seen in table II that utterances longer than two units in length were extremely rare prior to attainment of level-5 play and increased sharply in frequency during level-5 sessions.

Positional Patterns. Word combinations occurring at level-4 play were infrequent and exhibited so few specific patterns that a formal test of positional regularities proved unnecessary (table III). This would be expected if such early combinations were mediated by the relationship of each word to the given context, rather than based on a generative linguistic system.

After entry into level-5 play, positional patterns were observed in all subjects. Table IV presents the statistically significant positional patterns detected when *Braine's* [1976] criteria were applied to all two-word utterances produced by the children in the sessions described. These sessions were chosen to exemplify a number of patterns, although for each child some patterns were observed in earlier sessions.

These patterns accounted for approximately one third of each child's

Table II. Number of utterance types, two words or more in length

	Janis				Meri				Mira				Shanti				Tracy			
Session	2 words	3 words	4 words	> 4 words	2 words	3 words	4 words	> 4 words	2 words	3 words	4 words	> 4 words	2 words	3 words	4 words	> 4 words	2 words	3 words	4 words	> 4 words
1																	2			
2					1												1			
3	8					1			4								2			
4	7				5				13[a]				1	1			1	1		
5	4	1			3				3				3				3			
6	3	2			27[a]	2			26	4			0				5	2		
7	72[a,b]	25	7		66[b]	25	5	1	64[b]	30	10		14	3			4[a]	1		
8	59	37	13	1					73	37	10		68[a,b]	17	8		27	7	1	
9													59	32	16		27[b]	9	2	
10													67	37	15		51	16	0	
11													66	51	16	1				

[a] Session at which the child attained level-5 play.
[b] Session analyzed in table IV.

multi-word utterances produced in the session. The remaining combinations probably reflect a number of strategies, including the earlier context-dependent ordering which in some cases might parallel adult grammatical ordering (e.g., actor-action), some in which the child is 'groping' [*Braine*, 1976] for an appropriate order, and some exhibiting early acquisition of adult grammatical rules which override the earlier surface order rules. In the following paragraphs, in order to clarify the development of these combinations, the history of the patterns observed in each child's language samples will be noted, and results concerning utterances longer than two words will also be described – see tables III and IV for examples.

Janis. For Janis, 'a + x' had been used in previous sessions, and may have been learned earlier. She had not previously used the word 'it's', so 'It's + x' was probably new at session 7. Janis used few utterances longer than two words prior to this session, which was the month after entry into level-5 play. At this time she also showed a pattern of utterances beginning with 'I' including six exemplars, all of which were more than two words long. Janis' pattern of development suggests that she may have been emphasizing a 'gestalt' approach to language in which sentence frames are established and varied, rather than combinations being established on the basis of combining elements of earlier single-word vocabulary [*Nelson*, 1981].

Table III. Multiword utterances at level 4

Janis	Meri	Mira	Shanti	Tracy
Session 3	*Session 2*	*Session 3*	*Session 4*	*Session 5*
a + (baby, fish,	here baby	hi Mira	some more	iced tea
plate, shoe,	*Session 3*	sit down	*Session 5*	over here
toy, truck)	hey baby	where baby	get back	where baby
bye bye elephant	*Session 4*	orange juice	go in	*Session 6*
no toy	a bottle		I give it	baby down there
Session 4	Aunt Marcy		milk allgone	doll there
a mine	get it		*Session 6–0*	here go
a more	hey Ernie		*Session 7*	in here
bye bye banana	more cheese		a + (boy, cup,	oh baby
bye bye nose	*Session 5*		mommy)	oh there
more juice	all dirty		baby sit	over there
my baby	oh boy		baby there	*Session 7*
toy inere	what's that		blanket there	baby sleeping
Session 5			go night-night there	feed baby
a baby			night baby	here baby
a more			night-night there	here mommy
push it			one two	
there it is			one two three	
where piece			rock baby	
some more			swing wee	
Session 6			those two	
here it go			tickle it	
no more			tickle baby	
open it			two fish	
some more				

Meri. Comparison of Meri's patterns at session 7 with utterances in earlier sessions revealed that in session 6 (where level-5 play was first observed) she used the 'a + x' pattern, but there were too few utterances to establish significance. In contrast, 'baby' was used in both positions in the earlier session, rather than being confined to first position. Meri also exhibited a number of utterances of the form 'pronoun-verb-pronoun' (e.g., I get it, I do it) where either pronoun (but not both) could be replaced by a name (e.g., Mommy do it). These patterns have no apparent history in earlier sessions and the 'verbs' and 'pronouns' were never used as single words. Rather than true sentences, these seem to represent frames of limited mobility, anchored by the pronouns 'I' and/or 'it'. Similar patterns were reported by *Bloom* et al. [1975], *Braine* [1976], and *Nelson* [1973, 1981].

Mira. 'Mommy' was an extremely frequent single word for Mira (occurring 114 times, for example, at an early session). It can be seen (table III) that 'mommy' was in variable position in sessions 3, 4, and 5. By session 6, 2 months after planning was observed

Table IV. Two-word positional patterns[1] observed and examples of longer utterances

Janis – Session 7	Meri – Session 7	Mira – Session 7	Shanti – Session 8	Tracy – Session 9
It's+x (19/72)[2]	*a+x* (20/66)[2]	*Mommy+x* (31/64)[2]	*baby+x* (20/68)[2]	*Mommy+x* (9/27)[2]
It's+(baby's, blue,	a+(back, car, cup,	Mommy+(bang,	Baby+(blanket,	Mommy+(baby,
broken, doll,	fish, ride, shoes,	beads, bottle,	bottle, car, hat,	comb, do, there,
drinking, eating,	slipper)	button, dirt,	mine, on, shoes,	off on, phone,
fits, girl,	*baby+x*	elephant, finger,	turn)	this)
mommy, two,	baby+(car, mirror,	fish, hammer, hat,	*my+x*[4]	*Length > 2*
white)	mommy, phone,	hello, here, matter,	my+(baby, puzzle,	Mommy shoes on
a+x	pretty, there)	mine, mirror, more,	turn)	Mommy help me
a+(light, mommy,	*I+x*	off, play, pocket-	*Mommy+x*	Mommy one more
pink there,	I+(get, got, gots,	book, push, soup,	Mommy+(car, do,	Mommy pants off
sponge, 'w')	hammer, play, she,	there, tie, tired,	hat, here, peek-	I see it
Length > 2	shoes, can)	where, yes)	aboo, turn)	I do it
It's a boy	*Length > 2*	Reverse: (here,	*x+there*[4]	I get it
It's a mop	I close it	hello, ball, hold)	(hat, cow, on,	I sit
It's two baby	I do it	+Mommy	Shanti, window)	did it
	I get it	*here+x*[3]	+there	Put it on
	Mommy do it	here+(mirror, bottle,	*Length > 2*	
	I do beads	elephant, fish,	My baby elephant	
	I got this puzzle	soup)	My baby off	
	I did it all gone	*Length > 2*	Go in there	
	A baby phone	Mommy here a fish	It go there	
		Mommy here a mirror		
		here Mommy car		
		here Mommy finger		
		Mommy where a baby?		
		Mommy where soup?		

[1] Patterns are significant at the 0.05 level using a two-tailed binomial test except as noted.

[2] Proportion of total two-word types exemplifying these patterns.

[3] Based on a one-tailed test, alpha = 0.05.

[4] 'My' and 'there' patterns were significant only if imbedding patterns are considered as well as two-word patterns.

in play, the 'mommy + x' pattern was established. Session 7 exhibits the additional 'here + x' pattern.

Shanti. Utterances with 'baby' occurred with variable order prior to session 7. 'Mommy' and 'my' had not previously been used in combination. Utterances of the form 'x + there' occurred in session 6, prior to level-5 play, with too few exemplars to test for positional regularity.

Tracy. For Tracy a number of words appeared frequently enough in session 8 to allow evaluation of positional patterns. 'Baby', 'here', 'mommy' and 'no' were all used in combinations where they were equally likely to be found in first as last position. At session 9 the 'mommy' pattern remained the only positional pattern Tracy had developed. She also seemed to be developing a 'pronoun-verb-pronoun' pattern similar to that exemplified by Meri.

Discussion

Evidence has been presented for two levels of structural parallel between symbolic play and language: (1) the transition to combinations in both domains, and (2) the development of hierarchical symbolic structures allowing behaviors in play and language to be guided by prior mental acts. Since analogous nonlinguistic skills emerged close in time to similar language skills, mechanisms other than uniquely linguistic structures should account for the developments in both domains.

Concerning the first parallel, both level-4 play and the accompanying verbal combinations could result from the application of two new skills to symbolic contents: (1) the ability to combine symbols in relation to context [*McCall* et al., 1977], and (2) deferred imitation. *Werner and Kaplan* [1963] provided a rationale for children's initial limitation to single words and for the onset of verbal combinations, which is consistent with this interpretation. They suggested that children were originally limited to single word speech because each word referred to a global contextual tableau, rather than a set of interacting parts such as 'actors', 'objects', 'recipients', etc. As the symbolic capacity developed, the children would begin to differentiate these aspects of context and produce words with more delimited reference. Such words, since their meaning was now complementary rather than redundant, could be combined with reference to complementary aspects of context. Similarly, in language comprehension, language heard would be cognized by the child as composed of differentiated units, allowing the child to segment pairs of words from the language environment, and, through deferred imitation, produce such pairs later in appropriate contexts.

Deferred imitation refers to the repetition of a performance observed, at some time subsequent to the observation. According to *Piaget* [1962], deferred imitation marks the transition point between sensorimotor and representational abilities. *McCall* et al. [1977] observed imitation of novel sequences of behavior that had been presented to their 2-year-old subjects 24 h previously. The children varied and recombined elements of the complex behaviors, rather than imitating exactly. Hence sequences of words or actions previously observed could be reproduced either exactly or in an order imposed by the child. In the present study both verbal combinations learned as a unit and those involving unique constructions may reflect the influence of deferred imitation.

Early combinations in play reflect similar strategies. When the child applies the same action to several participants in succession, such as feeding self, mother, doll, it is apparent that the action 'feed' is now differentiated from any particular participant. In fact such play may reflect the child's statement to him- or herself that such multiple relationships are possible. Such ordered combinations as stirring in a dish, then feeding a doll may be based on exact deferred imitation, while combinations of actions such as feeding a doll, then combing its hair reflect the juxtaposition of two pretend acts (e.g., feed + comb) in a given context (doll play) and may also reflect a more varied use of deferred imitation.

The second structural parallel probably reflects the establishment of intentional symbolic relationships, a fundamental mental development which allows the child to cognize relations between symbols directly [*McCall* et al., 1977]. The effect of this skill on language would be to allow direct relationships between (1) linguistic symbols themselves and (2) language rules and lexical items. Reliance on context to support combinations would be reduced because of these new capabilities. In addition to rules of order, a general language spurt was apparent, close in time to the appearance of level-5 play. Frequency of speaking, MLU, and the number of different words used all accelerated sharply, and, for the first time, utterances longer than two words appeared. In addition *Nicolich and Raph* [1978] reported a rapid decline in immediate vocal imitation following entry into level-5 play for these same subjects.

An increase in play schemes and combinations was also observed at the transition to level 5 [*Nicolich*, 1977], suggesting a general facilitation of the symbolic function. In the present naturalistic study the number of play combinations remained too few to allow qualitative analyses of their structure such as that performed for language. However, *Fenson and Ramsay* [1981], who used modeling techniques to elicit pretend play sequences, reported a period of partial and unordered combinations, followed by ordered combinations. Similarly, *Corrigan* [1981], who used modeling to elicit both play and language sequences, found that the number of symbolic units expressed in play was related to the number of words imitated in utterances.

It may be that biological changes occurring late in the second year influence the symbolic capacity, leading to such uniquely human skills as complex language and planned symbolic play [*Wilson*, 1978]. It is notable that nonhuman primates learning nonvocal 'languages' do not exhibit the MLU spurt or structural development in language characteristic of human children [*Terrace* et al., 1979]. Rather, their communicative combinations remain unordered and context-dependent, like the play and language combinations observed in children at level-4 play.

Assuming, as the results presented here suggest, that both symbolic play and language are dependent on the development of underlying representational capacities, symbolic play may prove a useful tool for assessment and intervention with language-delayed children. For example, if 2 children whose language is below age level differ such that one exhibits age-appropriate symbolic play and other does not, this suggests both different etiologies for the language delay, and perhaps different strategies for intervention. In the first case language training can proceed directly based on the assumption that the symbolic system is appropriately developed. For the child exhibiting neither age-appropriate play nor language, perhaps cognitive intervention should supplement the language program. Training in symbolic play may prove an appropriate intervention vehicle. The strongest evidence for the basis of language and symbolic play on shared underlying structures would be the transfer to language of skills trained through play [*Bates and Snyder*, in press].

References

Bates, E.; Benigni, L.; Bretherton, I.; Camaioni, L.; Volterra, V.: From gesture to the first word: on cognitive and social pre-requisites; in Lewis, Rosenblum, Interaction, conversation and the development of language (Wiley, New York 1977).

Bates, E.; Benigni, L.; Bretherton, I.; Camaioni, L.; Volterra, V.: The emergence of symbols: cognition and communication in infancy (Academic Press, New York 1979).

Bates, E.; Camaioni, L.; Volterra, V.: The acquisition of performatives prior to speech. Merrill-Palmer Q. *21:* 205–226 (1975).

Bates, E.; Snyder, L.: The cognitive hypothesis in language development; in Uzgiris, McV.-Hunt, Research with scales of psychological development in infancy (University of Illinois Press, Champaign-Urbana, in press).

Belsky, J.; Most, R.K.: From exploration to play: a cross-sectional study of infant free play behavior. Devl Psychol. *17:* 630–639 (1981).

Bloom, L.: Language development: form and function in emerging grammars (MIT Press, Cambridge, Mass. 1970).

Bloom, L.: One word at a time: the use of single word utterances before syntax, p. 261 (Mouton, The Hague 1973).

Bloom, L.; Lahey, M.: Language development and language disorders (Wiley, New York 1978).

Bloom, L.; Lightbown, P.; Hood, L.: Structure and variation in child language. Monogr. Soc. Res. Child Dev. *40* (1975).

Braine, M.: Children's first word combinations. Monogr. Soc. Res. Child Dev. *41:* serial No. 164 (1976).

Branigan, G.: Some reasons why successive single word utterances are not. J. Child Lang. *6:* 411–423 (1979).

Brown, R.: A first language: the early stages (Harvard University Press, Cambridge, Mass. 1973).

Corrigan, R.: The control of actor-recipient relations in pretend play and language. Biennial Meeting of the Society for Research in Child Development, Boston 1981.

Crystal, D.: The analysis of intonation in young children; in Minifie, Lloyd, Communicative and cognitive development: early behavioral assessment (University Park Press, Baltimore 1978).

Dore, J.: Holophrases, speech acts and language universals. J. Child Lang. *2:* 21–39 (1975).

Dunn, J.; Wooding, C.: Play in the home and its implications for learning; in Tizard, Harvey, Biology of play (Lippincott, Philadelphia 1977).

Edwards, D.: Sensory-motor intelligence and semantic relations in early child grammar. Cognition *2:* 395–434 (1974).

Fein, G.: Imagination and play: some relationships in early development. Meeting of the American Psychological Association, Toronto 1978.

Fenson, L.; Ramsay, D.: Effects of modeling action sequences on the play of twelve, fifteen, and nineteen month old children. Child Dev. *52:* 1028–1036 (1981).

Fischer, K.: A theory of cognitive development: the control and construction of hierarchies of skills. Psychol. Rev. *87:* 477–531 (1980).

Howe, C.J.: The meanings of two-word utterances in the speech of young children. J. Child Lang. *3:* 29–47 (1976).

Jeffree, D.; McConkey, R.: Observation scheme for recording children's imaginative doll play. J. Child Psychol. Psychiat. allied Disc. *17:* 189–197 (1976).

Kahn, J.V.: Relationship of Piaget's sensorimotor period to language acquisition of profoundly retarded children. Am. J. ment. Defic. *6:* 640–643 (1975).

Largo, R.H.; Howard, J.A.: Developmental progression in play behavior of children between nine and thirty months. II. Spontaneous play and language development. Devl Med. Child Neur. *21:* 492–503 (1979).

Lowe, M.; Costello, A.: Manual for the symbolic play test; experimental ed. (NFER, London 1976).

Maratsos, M.P.; Chalkley, M.A.: The internal language of children's syntax: the ontogenesis and representation of syntactic categories; in Nelson, Children's language, vol. 2 (Gardner Press, New York 1980).

McCall, R.B.; Eichorn, D.H.; Hogarty, P.S.: Transitions in early mental development. Monogr. Soc. Res. Child Dev. *42:* serial No. 171 (1977).

McCall, R.; Parke, R.; Kavanaugh, R.: Imitation of live and televised models by children one to three years of age. Monogr. Soc. Res. Child Dev. *42:* serial No. 173 (1977).

McCune-Nicolich, L.: Toward symbolic functioning: structure of early pretend games and potential parallels with language. Child Dev. *52:* 785–797 (1981).

McNeill, D.: The development of language; in Mussen, Handbook of child psychology, vol. II (Wiley, New York 1970).

Nelson, K.: Structure and strategy in learning to talk. Monogr. Soc. Res. Child Dev. *38:* serial No. 149 (1973).

Nelson, K.: Individual differences in language development: implications for development and language. Devl Psychol. *17:* 170–187 (1981).

Nicolich, L.M.: Beyond sensorimotor intelligence: assessment of symbolic maturity through analysis of pretend play. Merrill-Palmer Q. *23:* 89–101 (1977).

Nicolich, L.M.; Raph, J.B.: Imitative language and symbolic maturity in the single word period. J. psycholinguist Res. *7:* 401–417 (1978).

Piaget, J.: Play, dreams and imitation (Norton, New York 1962).

Reynell, J.K.; Huntley, R.M.C.: New scales for the assessment of language development in young children. J. learn. Disabil. *4:* 549–557 (1971).

Rosenblatt, D.: Developmental trends in infant play; in Tizard, Harvey, Biology of play (Heinemann Medical Books, London 1977).

Sigman, M.; Ungerer, J.: Sensorimotor skills and language comprehension in autistic children (in preparation, 1980).

Steckol, K.; Leonard, L.: Sensorimotor development and pre-linguistic communication. J. Speech Hear. Res. (in press).

Terrace, H.S.; Petitto, L.A.; Sanders, R.J.; Dever, T.G.: Can an ape create a sentence? Science *206:* 891–902 (1979).

Werner, H.; Kaplan, B.: Symbol formation (Wiley, New York 1963).

Wilson, R.: Synchronies in mental development: an epigenetic perspective. Science *202:* 939–947 (1978).

Contr. hum. Dev., vol. 6, pp. 46–63 (Karger, Basel 1982)

Ways of Playing: Individual Differences in Imaginative Style

Dennie Wolf, Sharon Hya Grollman[1]
Harvard University, Cambridge, Mass., USA

Given the chance to watch several children playing, one of the sharper impressions is that of a marked, though hard-to-define, contrast in the way different children go about transforming the 'here-and-now' into what *Erikson* [1963] calls the 'microcosm of play' or what *Werner* termed 'an alternative reality' [*Franklin*, 1981]. Moreover, while any single child's play changes in length, intensity, theme and sophistication across time, there is often the impression of a kind of 'family resemblance' or similarity in style which persists throughout the changes brought by development and context. Both the contrasts and the continuity of such styles of playing are suggested by the following pairs of observations made of the same two children (in the observations contained in this chapter, *Je* refers to one subject; *An* refers to a second subject; *O.* refers to the adult observer).

Obs. 1a: At 1 : 0 the observer presents *Je* with a small toy tea set and several small dolls. *Je's* attention is attracted right away to a small plastic spoon. She places the spoon in her mouth and wanders about the room with the spoon protruding, mugging for her mother and the observer. *Je* stoops over to pick up a cup. She places the spoon in the cup, stirs it hard, and makes a 'mmmm' sound as if tasting something delicious. *Je* walks over to her mother, takes the spoon from her own mouth, and uses it to feed her mother repeatedly. Her mother enters the game, smacking her lips, saying 'mmmm' and asking for more. *Je* moves away and comes back with a small cup that she holds out to her mother, who obligingly drinks. *Je* then feeds her again. Upon walking away toward the window, *Je* encounters the dolls. She stoops and picks one up, drops it into a nearby chair where

[1] The longitudinal research reported in this paper has been supported through grants from the Carnegie and Spencer Foundations and the National Institutes of Education. We wish to thank the children and families involved in the study; *Pat McKernon, Shelley Rubin, Ann Smith* and *Jenny Shotwell* who were our co-investigators; and *Howard Gardner*, who commented on an earlier draft of this manuscript.

she feeds it from both the spoon and the cup. *Je* then takes the cup and, balancing it on her nose, turns to show her mother, who claps.

Obs. 1b: Presented with a small toy tea set and several small dolls, *An*, at 1:2, collects one doll, one cup and one spoon. She sits with them on her lap a moment, but then lifts them into the observer's lap. She is much more interested in the plates of various sizes that are spread out on the floor. She collects the four small ones first, making a neat stack of them. She then collects the four larger ones, also stacking them. *An* then nests the stack of smaller plates inside the set of larger ones. *An* places three remaining spoons on top of her stack; as she does so she makes smacking noises with her lips. She starts to offer the spoon to the observer and to her mother, simply holding it out toward each of them, but instead her attention returns to her previous interests and the process of unstacking and then rearranging the plates resumes.

Obs. 2a: At 3:5 *Je* is asked to play 'going on a boat trip'.

Je: 'Yeah, let's go in the boat. Oh, I see a wicked witch.'

O. and *Je* sit on the floor and pretend to look around.

O.: 'What else do you see?'

Je: 'I see two plates. They fell down... and there's some doors and they are getting ready to saw us.'

O.: 'Oh no.'

Je: 'We can go to Snow White's house.'

O.: 'Okay.'

O. and *Je* walk across the floor.

Je: 'Oh, no, don't go in there.' She approaches a small door in the hall and looks in. 'Oh-oh, she's sick. We better fix her up.' *Je* runs for her doctor kit and a different scenario ensues.

Obs. 2b: At 3:8 *An* is also asked to play 'going on a boat trip'. Along with *An*, *O.* settles on a cloth spread out on the living room floor.

O.: 'What do you see?'

An: 'I don't know. I want to get something else.' *An* leaves, coming back with dolls and books from her room.

O.: 'Did you want to read books, or just take them along?'

An: 'Take them with us. I better get a suitcase.' She does this. She unpacks numerous small toys from the suitcase. 'I'll throw these in the water 'cause all these are fishes.' She packs the dolls and books back into the suitcase. She then surveys the arrangement. She points to the rug area around the cloth where she sits. 'This is the water.' Touching the cloth, she says, 'This is the boat.'

The 2 children just described are, in many senses, well-matched. They share the same sex, age and background. They have been offered similar directions, in similar settings with the same adult as their partner in play. At each age, both children engage in the central project of symbolic play – the transformation of the 'here and now' into an alternative reality [*Bateson*, 1955; *Franklin*, 1981; *Freud*, 1959]. Nevertheless, the way in which each child carries out this project is distinctive. The first child, *Je*, uses words and gestures to create a fantasy narrative that unfolds more or less independent of the immediate physical environment. By comparison, *An's* symbolic play focuses quite closely on the concrete objects and spatial arrangements that make up her surroundings. The imaginative quotient of her play comes largely from her ability to 'mine' the attributes of her immediate physical environment in order to transform it from what it *is* to what it *could be*. In this way, *An* can 'see' that what *is* a blanket lying on a rug *could be* a boat floating on a river. Despite the similarities between children and situations, there appears to be a contrast in how each addresses the tasks inherent in symbolic play: *Je* elects to create a fantasy world *independent* of her physical surroundings while *An* constructs an imagined scene which is *dependent* on the careful observation of the objects and spaces around her.

Drawing up the contrast between *Je's* object-independent fantasy and *An's* object-dependent transformations leads to asking several questions: (1) How robust is this apparent contrast in the types of imaginative play? Do such differences exist outside this particular pair of children? If so, are such differences stable across changes in age, play sophistication, themes and materials? Most critically, what evidence is there that such contrasts in the conduct of play are more than the artifactual result of differences in individuals' maturity or sophistication in imaginative play? (2) How might strong evidence for developmentally-equivalent, but contrasting approaches to symbolic play affect our current model for the growth of an imaginative function? (3) How might such differences in play styles relate to previously established differences in cognitive style?

Based on earlier work concerning differences in individual play styles [*Gardner* et al., 1975; *Shotwell* et al., 1980; *Wolf and Gardner*, 1979], we propose that symbolic play can be conducted in at least two distinguishable formats: (a) as *object-independent fantasy play* in which the child creates an imaginary world by inventing events, roles and props 'out of thin air', and (b) as *object-dependent transformational play* in which the child creates an imaginary world by aptly transforming the objects and arrangements she actually finds around her. By demonstrating that preferences for a particular play style are independent of chronological age and an individual's level of development in play, we hope to indicate that play behaviors may evolve toward more than a single endpoint. In fact, we will suggest that the two play styles under discussion illustrate the broader possibility that developmentally-equivalent solutions to the same task can be constructed by individuals using contrasting strategies and following distinct cognitive routes [*Cole* et al., 1971; *Gilligan*, 1977].

Individual Differences in Play

Symbolization, or the representation of experience, is a complex undertaking. It requires that we make selections from personal history and understanding; choose among materials and grammatical options; elect to communicate with others or carry on an internal dialogue. Possibly because of this complexity, symbol use has consistently been thought of as revealing how different individuals make sense of their worlds [*Altschuler and Hattwick*, 1969; *Escalona*, 1968; *Fineman*, 1962; *Freud*, 1959; *Gould*, 1972; *Klinger*, 1969; *Peller*, 1954]. Among symbolic activities, play is perhaps the domain least constrained by societal rules and thus most full of options in the content and form of expression. As a result, play has consistently been used as a medium for examining the interaction between individuals, play themes [*Garvey and Berndt*, 1977; *Rubin* et al., 1976], social settings [*Jennings*, 1975; *Rubin* et al., 1976], and different types of imaginative play [*Dansky*, 1980; *Saltz*, 1978; *Saltz* et al., 1977; *Singer*, 1973].

Variety in Play's Endpoints

Despite the awareness of the complex interaction of individual players, materials and situations, there is at least one way in which the variety of play behaviors may have been underestimated. Virtually every major theorist who has taken an interest in play has described it as evolving from a dependence on objects towards an increasing independence from the prompts or supports which objects provide. This progression is evident in *Piaget's* [1961] observations of his children: he charted the evolution of Jacqueline's play from making pillows out of blankets and toys, through the transformation of objects to functionally and physically dissimilar referents (e.g., turning a shell into a cat), ending his description of her imaginative development with her ability to invent scenes, characters, and objects 'out of thin air'. A similar description emerges in *Freud's* [1959], *Vygotsky's* [1967], and *Singer's* [1973] separate discussions of the manner in which play evolves with age. This description of play as shifting from a dependence on objects to a relative independence from the object world has been extended in experimental and observational research in two ways. A first line of research has provided empirical details concerning the ages at which play shifts from object manipulation to object transformation, then to object-independent pantomime, and finally to internalized fantasy [*Chaillé*, 1978; *Lowe*, 1975; *Matthews*, 1977; *Singer*, 1973]. A second line of research has outlined the specific steps by which children are able to overlook the prototypical form and function of objects in the course of play. This work indicates that at first a child can only use an object out of its familiar context (as in drinking from a cup in play rather than at dinner). Subsequently, she may be able to overlook either the form or function of an object (as in using a cup as a hat for a doll). Only in a final stage of play substitutions can a child use an object to stand in for a referent which has both a dissimilar form and function (as in using a cup as if it were a toy car) [*Elder and Pederson*, 1978; *Fein*, 1975; *Jackowitz and Watson*, 1980]. In light of both types of evidence it seems appropriate to argue that object-independent play behaviors can be viewed as developmentally more sophisticated than object-dependent forms of imaginative play. In terms of judging children's cognitive maturity in play, it seems plausible to view object-dependent players, like *An*, as less sophisticated than object-independent peers, like *Je*.

Both steps in this argument may require re-examination. First, fantasy play may only appear in those cultural settings which actively encourage children to explore the subjective sides of experience. In settings where fantasy is discouraged, more elaborate and sophisticated forms of object-related play may characterize development [*Shotwell* et al., 1979]. Moreover, the second step of the argument overlooks the important distinction between players who are limited to object-dependent behaviors and players who, for reasons of interest or style, elect to exercise their imaginations chiefly, but not exclusively, on the objective side of experience [*Hudson*, 1966]. It is this second point that we want to examine in detail.

Evidence for Variety in Imaginative Behavior

There is, in fact, some support for the notion that individual children might exercise their capacity for imaginative behavior in distinctive ways. Existing research indicates that some children exhibit 'an imaginative predisposition' which leads them to symbolic play in which the frequency and depth of object-independent fantasy is greater than it is in their peers. Such children tend to play themes like Batman rather than 'going to the store'; they often report having imaginary companions and daydreams [*Hudson*, 1966; *Minuchin* et al., 1969; *Singer*, 1973]. In addition, *Matthews* [1977] has described two modes of fantasy transformation, material (making use of currently available props) and ideational (evoking nonpresent objects, roles or situations). Both modes are present in age-matched peers, varying in frequency with familiarity and with the sex of the players. Finally, *Winner* et al. [1979] report longitudinal evidence that individual children show preferences for the manner in which they transform objects in the service of make-believe during spontaneous play. One child may exploit the physical attributes of objects (e.g., calling a red plate an 'apple'), while a second child transforms an object to a very dissimilar referent through pantomime (e.g., using a small block as if it were a towel while pretending to take a bath).

Findings of this kind begin to suggest that even age-matched individuals vary in how they display their imaginative capacities. Moreover, such findings provide some support for the contrast between object-independent fantasy play and object-dependent transformational play which was outlined in the observations and discussion presented earlier. However, the more far-reaching hypothesis that equally sophisticated players display consistent but distinctive approaches to the task of make-believe demands both longitudinal data and measures which distinguish between the level of play behavior and the pattern of choices which typify its conduct.

Longitudinal Data

The observations, data, and conclusions presented here derive from an intensive, longitudinal study of early symbolic development conducted at Harvard Project Zero. In this study two separate cohorts of children were followed from their first birthday into their sixth year. In weekly home visits, children were observed both in free play and as they responded to a set of tasks designed to assess their abilities in a range of domains: symbolic play, story-telling, music, movement, number-use, two- and three-dimensional depiction. Transcripts of sessions were prepared from audiotapes, on-site observational notes and from video-taped sessions made at 4-month intervals. All observing and transcribing was done by two researchers, one acting as co-player, the other taking the part of an observer. The data presented in this chapter focus on the 4 girls from the first cohort of 5 subjects for whom data collection and analyses are currently complete. (The fifth subject in this cohort, a boy, consistently refused to engage in symbolic play. While this consistent pattern of refusal represents its own kind of individual difference in play, its inclusion here obscures the differences we want to highlight.)

The specific type of play considered here is sociodramatic play – the combination of gesture, language and object use which represents event sequences acted out by one or more players who assume various roles. The corpus of play analyzed for this study consisted of all instances of sociodramatic play performed by each of the 4 children between 1½ and 4½ years. These instances were drawn from a wide range of contexts: free play, children's insertion of play into other activities and tasks specifically designed to assess play abilities. Because we were examining the symbolic development of individual children, subjects' co-players were adult observers who entered into play whenever children requested their participation.

Contrast between Developmental and Stylistic Differences in Play

The concept of a *style* as a distinctive pattern of actions or attributes is a familiar notion; it turns up when we talk about an individual's 'personal style' or different living 'styles'. In discussions of art, music or writing, the concept is even more specific; it refers to the characteristic features of compositions which mark the works of individuals or schools *independent* of the content of those works [*Gardner*, 1970]. Thus, a viewer can recognize any number of Van Gogh paintings – whether portraits, still-lifes or landscapes – via the characteristic color schemes, forms and brush strokes. In the psychological realm, the concept of style rests on a similar distinction. Research in the area of cognitive style has sought to isolate the characteristic features of individuals' behavior which persist across a wide range of processes and tasks [*Witkin* et al., 1962, 1967]. Ideally, concepts of style are balanced; the description of any particular style should contain information about both the strengths and weaknesses of that particular approach [*Ward*, 1966, 1968].

Within developmental psychology, two additional criteria exist. First, stylistic differences must be conceptualized and shown to result from differences in the quality and not the developmental level of an individual's behavior. In more theoretical terms, there must be evidence that the proposed differences in style are independent of differences in cognitive maturity. Second, such individual differences in style must be shown to be stable across time. Such a demonstration is critical to showing that what appear to be stylistic differences are not the artifact of particular periods within development.

Designing the Investigation of Play Styles

The first step in this process was to establish a measure of the maturity of children's sociodramatic play such that we could construct developmentally-equivalent samples of each child's play at each of several ages. Based on earlier work concerning memory for events and stories [*Shank and*

Table I. Levels of narrative organization in play

Scheme level
At this level, children perform a single action or brief series of actions which re-enact motions, positions, and verbalizations associated with a single, small event. For example, a child holds a spoon to a doll's mouth as if feeding her.

Event script level
At this level, children perform at least two schemes which are part of the same process or part of achieving the same goal.

Simple events
This performance includes two to three different schemes, all of which are aimed at achieving a particular goal. For example, in a meal event, the child pours 'coffee' and offers it to her mother.

Contoured events
This performance involves at least four different schemes which are aimed at achieving a particular goal. For example, the child pours 'coffee', adds 'sugar', offers it to the experimenter while warning that it is 'hot'.

Episode level
At this level children perform at least two event scripts which are aimed at achieving a particular goal. The integration of scripts yields the outline of a situation, and each event that is enacted is flavored by the topic of that situation.

Simple episode
At least two simple events are enacted which are aimed at achieving a particular goal. For example, in a meal episode, the child enacts a cooking event in which she stirs the 'batter' and bakes it. Subsequently, the child enacts the event of serving the meal, in which she feeds the doll a piece of 'cake', then offers her 'milk'.

Contoured episode
At least two contoured events are enacted which are aimed at achieving a particular goal. For example, in a birthday party episode, the child enacts a cooking event in which she stirs the 'batter', adds 'sugar' and 'creamcheese', takes a spoonful for herself, then bakes it in the oven. The child then enacts a serving event as she gives her guests creamcheese cake and ice cream, while conversing with her 'friends' about what her doll did at her last birthday party.

Abelson, 1977; *Sutton-Smith* et al., 1976], we scored all instances of the children's sociodramatic play for the level of narrative organization or the ability to perform a sequence of events in a coherent and detailed way. The specific levels in the scoring system are presented in table I. Analysis of the coded data shows that all 4 children's play performances conform to the hypothesized sequences of levels. Thus, it appears that the level of narrative organization can serve as a broad indicator of the maturity of these children's sociodramatic play.

Table II. Rank-ordering of subjects based on age of acquisition[1] for levels of narrative organization in sociodramatic play (age is reported in weeks)

Scheme level	no discernible differences			
Event level				
Simple events	*Je* →	*Mi* →	*Ar* →	*An*
	66	68	82	98
Contoured events	*Ar* →	*Je* →	*An*	
	95	106	119	
	Mi →			
Episode level				
Simple episodes	*Mi* →	*Ar* →	*Je* →	*An*
	94	103	106	121
Contoured episodes	*Mi* →	*Je* →	*Ar* →	*An*
	109	122	149	187

[1] In our work we have defined the age of acquisition to be the second occasion when two raters agree that a child exhibits a particular level of narrative organization. For the purposes of this analysis, all highly ritualized or imitative sequences were eliminated from scoring. Two independent raters agreed on their assignment of play sequences to narrative levels in 87% of the instances.

The initial analysis of narrative organization provided additional important information: the 4 children pass through the successive levels at different rates. Table II presents a detailed picture of the rank order in which the 4 children attain each level. In summarizing these data, it is clear that 1 child, *Mi* is typically the first to move on to a more sophisticated level, whereas a second child, *An* is typically the last. The 2 children, *Ar* and *Je* appear to move forward at an intermediate rate.

This consistency in rank-ordering for their precocity clearly suggests that across time there are individuals who appear more skilled at, interested by or experienced in sociodramatic play. This finding provides an essential baseline for interpreting subjects' rank-order positions on subsequent measures of play. On measures where subjects' rank-ordering echoes that shown in table II, we have information on the correlates of precocity and possibly aptitude. Measures on which subjects rank differently provide important clues to those attributes of play which are independent of developmental level.

In order to test our hypothesis concerning two distinct but developmentally-equivalent styles of imagination, we constructed samples of age- and level-matched play performances for each subject. In designing these samples, we used overlapping rather than consecutive age periods, thereby increasing the amount of data within individual periods and increasing the robustness and accuracy of resulting characterizations [*Epstein*, 1980; *Mosteller* and *Tukey*, 1977]. The age ranges of the three age periods are: 1:6–2:9, 2:3–3:6, 3:0–4:6.

To assure a thorough match in our play samples, we assessed each child's performances, from each age period, for both the types of imaginative elements present and overall frequency with which such elements occurred. During each age period, each child gave evidence of the capacity to engage in both object-independent fantasy and object-dependent transformations. Moreover, if both types of make-believe are considered, there is no stable ordering of the 4 subjects which shows some individuals exhibiting a consistently higher level of imaginative content. With the exception of the earliest performances at the lowest level of narrative organization, the percent of an individual's performance given over to imaginative elements never differs by more than 15% across the 4 subjects. Despite the fact that the average frequency of imaginative elements climbs from under 10% to over 50% in these years, the children show remarkable inter-individual consistency. This indicates that whatever additional differences children exhibit in the imaginative quality of their play, these cannot be assumed to be the result of differences in a broad ability to get beyond 'the here-and-now'.

Specifying the Stylistic Differences in Play

By turning to a more precise analysis of the nature of imaginative content in play, it has been possible to provide evidence for the existence and endurance of the two styles of symbolic play suggested earlier: object-dependent fantasy and object-independent transformational play. In this analysis, all the imaginative elements in the age- and level-matched samples of play were isolated. Imaginative elements were defined as vocal or gestural schemes through which a child altered the pragmatic or actual constituents of the ongoing situation. Subsequently, these imaginative elements were broken down into those which were object-independent and those which were object-dependent. Object-independent instances of imagination were those that evoked nonpresent events, objects or persons (for example, a child pretending to make a cake performs a series of pinching and shaking gestures in the space above the bowl, saying 'salt, cinnamon and frosting'). Object-dependent instances were those that referred to actually present

Table III. Rank-ordering of subjects based on percentage of object-dependent imaginative verbalizations between 1:6 and 4:6

Scheme level (across all three age periods)	no discernible differences			
Event level				
Early events (1:6–2:9)	*Je*	*An*	*Mi* *Ar*	
	100 →	86 →	0	
Middle events (2:3–3:6)	*Mi* →	*An* →	*Je* *Ar*	
	100	82	33	
Late events (3:0–4:6)[1]	*An*		*Ar*	
	50	→	0	
Episode level				
Early episodes (1:6–2:9)	too few instances			
Middle episodes (2:3–3:6)	*An*	*Mi*	*Ar*	*Je*
	86 →	65 →	33 →	15
Late episodes (3:0–4:6)	*An*	*Mi*	*Ar*	*Je*
	53 →	51 →	17 →	4

[1] For this level and age period, only these 2 subjects have enough observations to merit a characterization of their performance.

events, object or persons (for example, a child pretending to make a cake, dropping a series of colored blocks into her bowl, saying, 'Now this one, this red one's a cherry, green for a green cherry').

As shown in table III, after 2:3, there is continuing evidence that the imaginative vocalizations of the children differ consistently in how object-dependent they are. Significantly, the rank-ordering of the children on this measure does not align with the earlier ranking of children for their precocity in narrative organization (table II). Moreover, from this same period, the frequency of object-dependent vocalizations is more similar within, as opposed to across the couples, *Ar-Je* and *Mi-An*. One interpretation of this pattern is that we are observing the clustering of individuals to a common approach as compared to the even distribution of children across the range of possible patterns of performance.

An examination of table IV indicates a similar pattern appears when nonverbal imaginative schemes are considered. The children in the couple *Mi-An* more frequently construct arrangements (e.g., laying out blocks in the pattern of a table-setting) and seek substitute items where an action

Table IV. Rank-ordering of subjects based on percentage of object-dependent, nonverbal imaginative elements between 1: 6 and 4: 6

Scheme level (across all age periods)	no discernible differences						
Event level							
Early events (1: 6–2: 9)	*An*		*Je*		*Mi*		*Ar*
	100	→	73	→	57	→	43
Middle events (2: 3–3: 6)	*Mi*		*An*		*Ar*		
	Je						
	100	→	87	→	43		
Late events (3: 0–4: 6)[1]	*An*						*Ar*
	66			→			37
Episode level							
Early episodes (1: 6–2: 9)	too few instances						
Middle episodes (2: 3–3: 6)	*Mi*		*An*		*Je*		*Ar*
	90	→	80	→	68	→	62
Late episodes (3: 0–4: 6)	*Mi*		*An*		*Ar*		*Je*
	61	→	59	→	40	→	36

[1] For this level and age period, only these 2 subjects have enough observations to merit a characterization of their performance.

typically requires a prop (e.g., rather than pantomiming the presence of batter in an empty bowl, these children prefer to place blocks there to be stirred). The couple *Ar-Je* finds pointing out entirely imaginary objects and pantomime both easy and acceptable. This contrast emerges somewhat later than in vocalizations, possibly because skills like pantomime and the reconstruction of spatial arrangements appear later than their language counterparts.

The picture of these two play styles can be filled out descriptively. In this more detailed view, it becomes clear that the play of *An* and *Mi* (the object-dependent subjects) is an activity which is deeply observant of objects since it takes off from, rather than remaining tied to, the contents of the environment. *Mi* treats red beads as pitted cherries; *An* uses a jaggedly-shaped piece of felt as if it were waves at the edge of the rug which serves as an ocean. This skill is hardly confined to objects. *An* and *Mi* frequently construct play terrains and rigorously maintain the novel identities that they assign to familiar objects. *Mi*, for example, turns the throw rugs in her living room into islands with the floor as ocean and the furniture as boats and houses. Throughout a 2-hour observation session, even when block-building and singing, she continues to hop from one rug to the next, saying she 'needs to stay dry'. As this last example implies, once such children make transformations they are likely to conserve them. *An*, having used one cylinder as a nail while playing carpenter, goes on to address each new, similarly-sized cylinder as if it, too, were a nail. In the context of sociodramatic play, this respect for or interest in objects has a somewhat conservative side. When other players offer novel names or uses for an object, *An* or *Mi* may refuse to adopt these, seeking what is a 'better' substitute. At one point, *Mi* refuses to use a long block as a knife, preferring to run and get a tinker toy stick. These 'rules' governing denotation are most pronounced when other players perform bits of fantasy, as when *An* rejects an empty toy plate as 'a piece of cake' until she has placed a small rectangular block on it. Perhaps the most striking evidence of these children's curiosity about and interest in the object world appears in situations where the properties or workings of an item interrupt the pretense entirely, turning it to investigation and experimentation [*Berlyne*, 1960, 1970; *Hutt*, 1979]. At a simple level this is evident in the earliest observation of *An*, where the matching and stacking of plates takes over from the dinner scenario.

Sociodramatic play often includes elements which are not particularly imaginative. In the course of playing 'dinnertime' a child may stop pretending in order to count the plates or ask 'How come this one is broken?' Observations of these breaks in make-believe suggest that the individual differences found in imaginative behaviors may have parallels in other domains. Currently, it appears that the sociodramatic play of object-dependent children is full of such breaks. At all levels and ages, these children frequently break off the scenario they are playing out in order to pay rapt attention to some present object or ongoing event that captures their attention. Even as late as 4:0, object-dependent children are easily distracted from the story component of their play by the possibility of experimenting with the number, arrangement and physical properties of the props at hand. (One such child left off pretending to pour tea in favor of stacking the cups and saucers into a sort of 'leaning tower', using a spoon balanced in the spout to experiment with different strategies of toppling the tower.)

Object-independent children exhibit different play behaviors. Their play can be so invulnerable to the 'real world' that they scoop up actual events and objects, assimilating them to the flow of play sequences. *Je*, in the middle of playing out an episode from the story of Snow White, spies a toy doctor kit, which captures her attention. Adeptly, she moves the narrative to a point where the stethoscope and hypodermic needle can be absorbed without fracturing the continuity of the story: 'Snow White isn't feeling too good, so say she needed to go and see the doctor.' On another occasion, during a trip scene, a noon whistle blows outside. *Je* assimilates the sound: 'Oh, no, that's the lion. We have to be very careful.' The play rules these children establish, pursue and enforce have to do with the maintenance of fantasy – in particular the carrying-out of assumed roles and sustaining make-believe. It is sometimes hard to get them to leave pretense. *Ar*, upon being asked to tell an oral story refuses. When the request is repeated, she dodges it by continuing an earlier occurring bit of pretense with a doll: 'I'm sorry. But it's too late for a story now. You have to go to bed. Right now, okay?'

In addition, object-independent children are much less concerned with the appropriateness and system behind object substitutions in play. They are capable of making outlandish substitutions, apparently because of the narrative motivation and dramatic pantomime surrounding the substitution.

Thus, *Ar* can use a tiny cube block for a bath towel by shimmying and shivering as she rubs it over the surface of her body. In a similar vein, object substitutions have no binding force for such children. *Je*, in the course of several minutes of play uses the same clothespin for a spoon, a pot handle, and a knife as the changing course of her scenario demands new props.

Individual Differences Outside Play

Styles of Symbol Use

In previous work [*Gardner* et al., 1975; *Shotwell* et al., 1980; *Wolf and Gardner*, 1979], we have hypothesized the possibility of at least two broad approaches to experience which may have significant effects for the course and content of early symbolic development. The two approaches or styles were: (a) the patterner who exhibits a sensitivity to the objective dimensions of experience like quantity, shape, size and color. As a result, a patterner excells in visual-spatial tasks and in the creation of designs and systems. Individuals of this bent frequently display a complementary reticence, if not a disability, in domains which demand the construction and exploration of more social and subjective forms of experience like discussion, story-telling, and pure fantasy; (b) the dramatist who is alive to many of the personal and social dimensions of experience, like roles, attitudes and strategies. Consequently, dramatists shine in games, sociodramatic play, arguments and negotiations. However, these individuals typically grow bored and frustrated, performing poorly when asked to pursue highly organized tasks which demand close attention to the properties of objects (e.g., puzzles, counting, classification, etc.). The findings reported here concerning two different orientations to the object world present an empirical picture of how the predilections of patterners and dramatists might affect behavior in a particular domain.

Clearly, there is also the question of how these findings relate to other investigations of cognitive style. Perhaps the clearest connections arise in the context of other studies of individual differences in early symbolization. *Matthews*' [1977] work on modes of transformation in play points out two modes of make-believe, material and ideational, which directly parallel our concepts of object-dependent and object-independent play. *Matthews* [1977] indicates that individuals may vary in the extent to which they depend on either of these modes of transformation. Similarly, *Nelson's* [1973] research on the content of early vocabularies has shown that it is possible to distinguish between referential and expressive speakers, whose first 50 words focus either on naming the contents of the immediate environment or in learning terms that figure prominently in social interactions (e.g., 'Thank you').

Structural Effects of Patterns of Interest

The content of symbolic activities may be indicative of fundamental differences in what attracts and holds individual children's attention. If so, the questions can be asked, 'Do such differences have consequences for patterns of activity and skill profiles outside of such clearly expressive areas like play and language use?'

Based on the ongoing analysis of the longitudinal data, we are building a picture of additional behaviors that correlate with either the objective orientation of patterners or the subjective orientation of dramatists. An analysis of free-play choices shows that patterners (who are object-dependent players) prefer items like blocks, markers and clay to items that imply less explicit attention to object attributes – like costumes. The inverse appears to be true of dramatists (who are object-independent players). Moreover, when children convert materials from typical to novel uses, it appears their conversions follow the pattern of preference evident in free play. Thus, an object-dependent child might take the teapot and side-step its use as a prop in sociodramatic play, opting to experiment with pouring liquids from it. Research concerning the consequences or even the correlations between spontaneous patterns of interest and skill profiles is rare. However, there is some evidence from *Jennings* [1975] that there are both clear person – versus object – orientations and that these predilections may correlate with either social or object-related problem-solving skills.

Broad Cognitive Styles

The work on individual differences in early symbolization or patterns of interest points to contrasts in either the structure or the content of behavior in early childhood. However, the most detailed research on differences concerns the manner in which children typically approach tasks. *Kagan* and his associates have described two such broad cognitive styles, impulsivity and reflectivity [*Kagan*, 1965, 1966; *Kagan and Kogan*, 1970], while *Witkin* et al. [1962, 1967] have outlined the characteristics of field-dependent and field-independent individuals. Thus, during the preschool years, there is evidence that children's behavior shows individually consistent patterns of approach, structure and content. Currently, what we lack is a synthesis. Intuitively, it seems plausible that patterners might exhibit object orientations and a reflective or even field-independent approach given their absorption with the details of shape, color, number and design. Contrastingly, dramatists may be strongly oriented to the world of people and given to impulsivity or field dependence, due to their desire to keep pace and be 'in tune' with the interpersonal world. Such intuitions require investigation, however.

Conclusion

Given the homogeneity of our sample, its small size, the length and intensity of interactions between children and observers, we have to wonder if all, or even most, preschool children would exhibit the specific styles of imaginative play or the broader predilections for the objective versus subjective sides of experience that we have proposed. The generality with which object-dependent and object-independent play occurs needs to be examined as a part of the larger process of examining the interaction between common developmental tasks and the specific individuals who negotiate them. Despite the accruing evidence that young children maintain characteristic approaches, structures and contents in their behavioral repertoires, we are still in search of a theory that would predict the interrelatedness or independence of these traits. Pursuing such a theory seems vital as it may lead toward understanding how individuals of different cognitive styles, sexes or cultures arrive at distinctive, though equivalent, solutions to the issues in human development.

References

Altschuler, R.; Hattwick, L.: Painting and personality (University of Chicago Press, Chicago 1969).

Bateson, G.: A theory of play and fantasy. Psychiat. Res. Rep. *2:* 39–51 (1955).

Berlyne, D.E.: Conflict, arousal and curiosity (McGraw-Hill, New York 1960).

Berlyne, D.: Laughter, humor and play; in Lindzey, Aronson, The handbook of social psychology; 2nd ed., vol. 3, pp. 795–852 (Addison-Wesley, Reading 1970).

Chaillé, C.: The child's conceptions of play, pretending and toys: sequences and structural parallels. Human. Dev, *21:* 201–210 (1978).

Cole, M.; Gay, J.; Glick, J.A.; Sharp, D.W.: The cultural context of learning and thinking (Basic Books, New York 1971).

Dansky, J.: Make-believe: a mediator of the relationship between play and associative fluency. Child Dev. *51:* 576–579 (1980).

Elder, J.L.; Pederson, D.R.: Preschool children's use of objects in symbolic play. Child Dev. *49:* 500–504 (1978).

Epstein, S.: The stability of behavior. II. Implications for psychological research. Am. Psychol. *35:* 790–806 (1980).

Erikson, E.H.: Childhood and society (Norton, New York 1963).

Escalona, S.K.: The roots of individuality (Basic Books, New York 1968).

Fein, G.G.: A transformational analysis of pretending. Devl Psychol. *11:* 291–296 (1975).

Fineman, J.: Observations on the development of imaginative play in early childhood. Child Psychiat. *1:* 167–181 (1962).

Franklin, M.: Object, action, and language in symbolic play. 1st Bienn. Conf. of the Heinz Werner Institute of Developmental Psychology, Worcester 1981.

Freud, S.: Creative writers and daydreaming; in Strachey, The standard edition of the complete psychological works of Sigmund Freud; vol. IX, pp. 141–154 (Hogarth, London 1959).

Gardner, H.: Children's sensitivity to painting styles. Child Dev. *41:* 813–821 (1970).

Gardner, H.; Wolf, D.; Smith, A.: Artistic symbols in early childhood. N.Y. Univ. Q. *6:* 13–21 (1975).

Garvey, C.; Berndt, R.: Organization of pretend play. Annu. Meet. of the American Psychological Association, Chicago 1977.

Gilligan, C.: In a different voice: women's conception of the self and of morality. Harvard educ. Rev. *47:* 481–517 (1977).

Gould, R.: Child studies through fantasy (Quadrangle Press, New York 1972).

Hudson, L.: Contrary imaginations (Schocken, New York 1966).

Hutt, C.: Exploration and play; in Sutton-Smith, Play and learning, pp. 231–251 (Gardner Press, New York 1979).

Jackowitz, E.; Watson, M.: Development of object transformations in early pretend play. Devl Psychol. *16:* 543–549 (1980).

Jennings, K.D.: People vs. object orientation, social behavior, and intellectual abilities in pre-school children. Devl Psychol. *1:* 511–519 (1975).

Kagan, J.: Impulsive and reflective children: significance of conceptual tempo; in Krumboltz, Learning and the educational process, pp. 133–161 (Rand McNally, Chicago 1965).

Kagan, J.: Reflection – impulsivity: the generality and dynamics of conceptual tempo. J. abnorm. Psychol. *71:* 17–24 (1966).

Kagan, J.; Kogan, N.: Individual variation in cognitive processes; in Mussen, Handbook of child psychology, vol. 1, pp. 1273–1365 (Wiley, New York 1970).

Klinger, E.: Development of imaginative behavior: implications of play for a theory of fantasy. Psychol. Bull. *72:* 277–298 (1969).

Lowe, M.: Trends in the development of representational play in infants from one to three years: an observational study. J. Child Psychol. Psychiat. *16:* 33–47 (1975).

Matthews, W.S.: Modes of transformation in the initiation of fantasy play. Devl Psychol. *13:* 211–216 (1977).

Minuchin, P.; Biber, B.; Shapiro, E.; Zimiles, H.: The psychological impact of school experience (Basic Books, New York 1969).

Mosteller, F.; Tukey, J.W.: Data analysis and regression (Addison-Wesley, Reading 1977).

Nelson, K.: Structure and strategy in learning to talk. Monogr. Soc. Res. Child Dev. *38:* serial No. 141 (1973).

Peller, L.: Libidinal phases, ego development and play. Psychoanal. Study Child *9:* 178–198 (1954).

Piaget, J.: Play, dreams and imitation (Norton, New York 1961).

Rubin, K.H.; Maioni, T.L.; Hornung, M.: Free play behaviors in middle and lower class preschoolers: Parten and Piaget revisited. Child Dev. *47:* 414–419 (1976).

Saltz, E.: Stimulating imaginative play: some cognitive effects on pre-schoolers. Annu. Meet. of the American Psychological Association, Toronto 1978.

Saltz, E.; Dixon, D.; Johnson, J.: Training disadvantaged preschoolers on various fantasy activities: effects on cognitive functioning and impulse control. Child Dev. *48:* 367–380 (1977).

Shank, R.; Abelson, R.: Scripts, plans, goals and understanding (Lawrence Erlbaum Ass., Hillsdale 1977).

Shotwell, J.; Wolf, D.; Gardner, H.: Exploring early symbolization: styles of achievement; in Sutton-Smith, Playing and learning, pp. 126–157 (Gardner Press, New York 1979).

Shotwell, J.; Wolf, D.; Gardner, H.: Styles of achievement in early symbolization; in Foster, Brandes, Symbol as sense: new approaches to the analysis of meaning, pp. 115–199 (Academic Press, New York 1980).

Singer, J.L.: The child's world of make-believe (Academic Press, New York 1973).

Sutton-Smith, B.; Botvin, G.; Mahony, D.: Developmental structures in fantasy narratives. Hum. Dev. *9:* 1–3 (1976).

Vygotsky, L.: Play and the role of mental development of the child. Soviet Psychol. *5 (3):* 6–18 (1967).

Ward, W.C.: Creativity and impulsivity in kindergarten children; doct. diss. Duke Univ. (1966).

Ward, W.C.: Reflection-impulsivity in kindergarten children. Child Dev. *39:* 867–874 (1968).

Winner, E.; McCarthy, M.; Kleinman, S.; Gardner, H.: First metaphors. New Direct. Child Dev. *1:* 29–41 (1979).

Witkin, H.A.; Dye, R.B.; Paterson, H.F.; Goodenough, D.R.; Karp, S.A.: Psychological differentiation (Wiley, New York 1962).

Witkin, H.A.; Goodenough, D.R.; Karp, S.A.: Stability of cognitive style from childhood to young adulthood. J. soc. Psychol. *1:* 291–300 (1967).

Wolf, D.; Gardner, H.: Style and sequence in early symbolic play; in Smith, Franklin, Early symbolization, pp. 117–138 (Erlbaum, Hillsdale 1979).

Contr. hum. Dev., vol. 6, pp. 64–78 (Karger, Basel 1982)

Play and Divergent Thinking

Debra J. Pepler

Erindale College, University of Toronto, Mississauga, Ont., Canada

There is a widespread belief among developmental psychologists and educators that play is a primary medium through which children develop cognitive skills, particularly those skills related to creativity or divergent thinking [*Bruner*, 1974; *Sutton-Smith*, 1967, 1968]. The purpose of this chapter is to examine the link between play and creativity. To establish a framework, I will first review the research that demonstrates a relationship between play and creativity and the research that shows play to facilitate divergent thinking. Second, I will attempt to identify the behaviors, processes and factors of the play experience that mediate the relationship between play and creativity. In doing so, I will consider both the theoretical perspectives concerning the processes in play that contribute to creativity and the empirical evidence relating individual and situational factors in play to creative performance.

The Relationship between Play and Creativity

Interest in the contribution of play to creativity has stemmed primarily from research that demonstrated a correlation between several play behaviors and divergent thinking. *Lieberman* [1965] was among the first to examine this relationship. She asked kindergarten teachers to rate their students on five components of playfulness: physical spontaneity; social spontaneity and cognitive spontaneity; manifest joy, and sense of humor. *Lieberman* [1965] found strong correlations between these playfulness traits and three divergent thinking factors: ideational fluency (the ability to generate a large number of responses that meet a certain criterion); spontaneous flexibility (the ability and disposition to vary responses), and originality (the ability to generate unique responses).

Following *Lieberman's* [1965] work, *Sutton-Smith* [1968] presented kindergarten boys and girls with male and female sex-typed toys and asked them for alternate uses for these toys. The boys and girls were presumed to be equally familiar with toys associated with each sex, but to have differential play experiences with same-sex and opposite-sex toys. The relationship between play experiences and divergent thinking was demonstrated in that boys and girls gave more unique responses for the toys ascribed to their own sex. *Sutton-Smith* [1968] suggested that the novel responses associated with an object during play contributed to the creativity of responses regarding that object in the task situation.

Johnson [1976] examined the relation of divergent thinking test scores with social and nonsocial make-believe play of 3- to 5-year-old children. The children were observed during free play at nursery school and scored for the type of fantasy play they engaged in. The children were given a multiple use task and a story completion task as measures of divergent thinking. *Johnson* [1976] found that only social fantasy play, and not nonsocial fantasy play, was related to performance on the divergent tasks. He suggested that the factor common to both divergent thinking and social fantasy play might be ideational fluency.

Singer and Rummo [1973] also examined the relationships between divergent thinking, as measured by ideational fluency, and creativity and playfulness in kindergarten children. They found that highly creative boys were more communicative, curious, humorous, playful, and expressive. For girls, none of the playfulness measures was related to creativity alone, but they interacted with measures of IQ. These findings suggested that, for boys at least, there is a relation between styles of play and divergent thinking.

Hutt and Bhavnani [1976] assessed children who had taken part in a prior study of exploration with a novel toy. On the basis of the first study, these 3- to 5-year-old children were categorized as: (1) nonexplorers who looked at a toy, but did not investigate it in any way; (2) explorers who actively investigated the toy, but did not go beyond specific exploration, and (3) inventive explorers who investigated the new toy and then used it in imaginative ways as in diversive exploration. There was a sex difference in group membership, with girls overrepresented as nonexplorers and boys overrepresented as inventive explorers. A test of divergent thinking was given to these children. The results indicated that inventive play was positively correlated with the measures of divergent thinking, but primarily for boys.

In the aforementioned studies a variety of play behaviors was related to divergent problem-solving skills. These were: playfulness; manipulating objects; exploring object properties; exhibiting novel responses, and playing symbolically with objects. The extant research also suggests that play and divergent thinking may have common underlying factors such as ideational fluency.

The weakness of these and other correlational studies, as *Hutt* [1982] cautioned, is that it is impossible to determine whether play experiences cause developmental change or whether the link between play and creativity is simply the result of a similar cognitive style. If, in fact, play enhances divergent problem-solving performance, it is important to identify the variables of the play experience that relate to creativity. The direction and nature of this association will be examined in more detail in the next section.

The Effects of Play on Creativity

Researchers who investigate the effects of play on creativity, typically present children with objects during play or nonplay sessions and subsequently test them on divergent thinking tasks which measure the number and originality of responses. One of the first such studies was conducted by *Dansky and Silverman* [1973], who assigned children, aged 4–6 years, to one of three conditions: a play condition, an imitation condition, and a neutral condition, in which the children colored. The children were given 10 min of play, imitation or coloring and tested immediately thereafter on the Alternate Uses Task. There were no differences among the groups on standard responses (referring to a use for which the object was designed). However, the children in the play condition were superior to the imitation and control groups on the number of nonstandard responses for the objects (any other nonredundant response). In a discussion of the effects of play on performance on the Alternate Uses Task, *Dansky and Silverman* [1973] noted that some of the responses of the children in the play group reflected their activities with the objects during play; however, not all of the responses could be related to previous play behaviors. In addition, children who were in the play condition made more use of environmental cues in their search for responses to the task. The authors suggested that the children who had played may have come into the testing situation with a more playful attitude, thereby approaching the divergent task with more flexibility, curiosity, spontaneity, and interest.

In a subsequent study, *Dansky and Silverman* [1975] tested the generality of the effect of play on associative fluency. Children were exposed to one set of materials in play, imitation, or intellectual task condition and were then asked the alternate uses for another set of materials. The children in the play condition produced significantly more standard and nonstandard uses than either the imitation or the intellectual task groups, even though the objects had not been available during play. *Dansky and Silverman* [1975, p. 104] concluded that the results of their two studies 'lend strong support to the notion that play creates a set, or attitude, to generate associations to a variety of objects whether or not these objects are encountered during play activity'.

Li [1978] conducted a study to replicate and extend the research of *Dansky and Silverman* [1973, 1975] by examining two factors that might link play experience and superior performance on the Alternate Uses Task. As in *Dansky and Silverman's* [1975] study, *Li* [1978] included an unfamiliar object in the posttests to assess whether a playful attitude results in a general lowering of the threshold for novel association. In other words, the play children were expected to give more novel associations for an object, even if it had not been encountered in play. The second question that *Li* [1978] examined was whether the make-believe aspect of play was the link to divergent thinking. To investigate this possibility, a make-believe group was included; they were asked to think about the materials in a pretend way. Apart from these two additions, the procedures were similar to those of *Dansky and Silverman* [1973, 1975]. Children aged 4 and 5 years were randomly assigned to one of four groups: free play, make-believe play, imitation and control. The children were given 10 min of individual experience according to their group membership. Immediately thereafter, the Alternate Uses Task was administered.

The results of this study were unclear in terms of the superiority of free play versus directed make-believe play. The make-believe subjects gave more nonstandard responses for the unfamiliar item. For one of the familiar items both the free play and make-believe play subjects were superior to the imitation and control subjects. The author concluded that the direction of make-believe play may have a greater facilitating effect on divergent thinking than free play; however, this was only shown to be true for the unfamiliar object. Although these findings lend support to the relationship between play and divergent thinking, they do not clearly identify the specific elements in play that facilitate creativity.

In a recent study, *Dansky* [1980a] also examined the role of make-believe or fantasy as a primary factor in play contributing to creativity. Prior to treatment, preschool subjects were categorized during free play as either 'players' (who displayed make-believe) or 'nonplayers'. They were assigned to one of three conditions: free play, imitation, and convergent problem-solving. After a 10-min treatment session, the children were asked to name the uses for unfamiliar objects. *Dansky* [1980a] found that the beneficial effects of free play on fluency in a creativity task were limited to those children who typically engaged in make-believe play in the classroom. Based on this and earlier findings, *Dansky* [1980a] postulated that certain cognitive processes that are involved in make-believe or fantasy play, such as free association and symbolic thinking, are similar to those involved in divergent thinking.

An effect of play on divergent thinking was also found in two studies that *Pepler* [1979] and *Pepler and Ross* [1981] conducted on play and problem-solving. In the first study 3- and 4-year-old children were assigned to four conditions: (1) play with convergent materials, (2) play with divergent materials, (3) observe convergent activity, and (4) observe divergent activity. The play materials, five sets of nine pieces which fit into five formboards, could be used as puzzles (convergent activity) or play blocks (divergent activity). Children in the convergent play condition played with the pieces and the formboards; children in the divergent play condition played with only the pieces. The control groups observed the experimenter engaging in convergent or divergent activity. All children participated individually in three 10-min sessions and were given a battery of divergent problem-solving tasks after the third session. Children who had divergent play experiences gave more unique responses on a divergent thinking task than all other groups.

The second study was similar to the first except that a nonplay control replaced the observe conditions and the divergent thinking tasks were modified. In this study the divergent group again gave more unique responses than the other groups. These findings indicate that children who had divergent play experiences were more imaginative in their responses to divergent thinking tasks, suggesting that it is not play per se, but play with unstructured play materials that contributes to creativity.

In summary, there is considerable support for the effect of play on creative performance. Taken together, these studies indicate that children given play experiences perform better on divergent thinking tasks than children with imitation, intellectual, convergent, or neutral experiences. Several processes by which play may contribute to creativity are suggested by the research. First, there may be a generalized transfer of a playful attitude or a flexible response set from the play to problem-solving situations. Hence children with play experiences may be more flexible, curious, spontaneous and interested in the task [*Dansky and Silverman*, 1973, 1975]. Second, there may be a more specific transfer of novel responses generated by investigation and experimentation in play. Children with play experiences were found to make more use of previous play activities to generate responses on a divergent thinking task [*Dansky and Silverman*, 1973]. Third, symbolic activity in play may facilitate creative performance. Although symbolic activity was not measured systematically during treatment sessions, the data suggest that those children who benefited most from play experience were those whose play likely included make-believe elements. It has been suggested that the cognitive skill of shifting one's thinking from the concrete to abstract during play may be similar to the skill required to generate a variety of novel responses on a divergent thinking task [*Johnson*, 1976; *Singer and Rummo*, 1973].

These processes presumed to mediate the link between play and creativity may also interact with individual and situational factors. For example, some research indicates that children with a predisposition for make-believe play [*Dansky*, 1980a] or inventive exploration [*Hutt and Bhavnani*, 1976] tend to be more creative. Other research suggests that characteristics of the play experience, such as the structure of the play materials [*Pepler*, 1979; *Pulaski*, 1973] or social interaction [*Johnson*, 1976], affect subsequent divergent problem-solving performance. In order to examine these processes underlying the link between play and creativity, I will now consider the theories that purport to explain the influence of play on development. This presentation will be followed by a more detailed examination of the individual and situational factors relating play to creativity.

Theories on Play and Development

An examination of the major theories of play yields three common themes concerning the ways that play contributes to the development of divergent problem-solving skills. These are: (1) play as investigation, (2) experimentation and flexibility in play, and (3) facilitating the transition from concrete to abstract thought through play. The theories related to each of these themes will be reviewed in order to specify the way in which they account for the contributions of play to divergent thinking.

Play as Investigation

First, investigation or exploration in play is presumed to contribute to development. There is a controversy throughout the literature about the distinction between play and exploration, and whether exploration is, in fact, a form of play. Since the intent of this chapter is not to define play, but to examine specific play behaviors and processes that relate to divergent thinking, exploration will be included in this discussion of the means by which play contributes to development.

Two types of exploration have been identified, specific and diversive [*Hutt*, 1982]. Specific exploration is seen when a child is confronted with a novel object. It has the intent of asking, 'What is this and what can it do?' [*Berlyne*, 1965] and applies to this theme of play as investigation. Diversive exploration has the intent of asking, 'What can I do with this object?' [*Hutt*, 1982] and relates to the next theme. Specific exploration is characterized by visual investigation, active examination, manipulation and a prolonged attention to the object and activities with it [*Berlyne*, 1965; *Hutt*, 1982; *Piaget*, 1962]. There is considerable evidence that through specific exploration or the investigation of novel objects the child develops a fuller understanding of these objects [*Weisler and McCall*, 1976]. Specific exploration, as such, would likely be beneficial to subsequent problem-solving with the same objects by providing the child with an initial understanding of the objects.

Experimentation and Flexibility in Play

The second mechanism through which play contributes to development is by the experimental and flexible nature of play activities. Once the child has mastered a skill or discovered the properties of an object, she or he begins to experiment actively with the action or object. This experimentation in play purportedly contributes to variability [*Sutton-Smith*, 1975] and flexibility [*Bruner*, 1973] in the child's responses.

Experimentation in play has been described as a more advanced activity following specific investigation of an object. *Hutt* [1982] described this as diversive exploration when the child begins to vary his or her responses to an object. In contrast to specific exploration in which the child examines the properties of an object, in diversive exploration the child investigates different ways of using the object. *Hutt* [1982] observed that diversive exploration is characterized by a more relaxed and varied approach to the objects of play. It involves trial and error and the chance combinations of responses [*Piaget*, 1962] and is a form of 'variation-seeking' with an object and a child's own behaviors [*Sutton-Smith*, 1975]. *Bruner* [1973] described the experimental mechanism in play as combinatorial flexibility in which the child's skills form subroutines which are then subjected to experimentation and later incorporated into more complex activities. The benefit of this experimental mechanism in play is that it provides a broad repertoire of skills and responses and perhaps a flexible set that can be evoked to more effectively approach a divergent thinking task.

Facilitating the Transition from Concrete to Abstract Thought

Several major theorists postulated that play facilitates the transition from concrete to abstract thought [*Piaget*, 1962; *Smilansky*, 1968; *Vygotsky*, 1976]. In *Piaget's* [1962] terms, the transition is from sensorimotor schemes to conceptual schemes. Representation occurs in play when a symbol (signifier) takes on the meaning of an object (signified). According to *Piaget* [1962], the meanings of symbols are, in part, evoked through assimilation which is the dominant element in play. Hence the symbolic representations that are produced in play (for example, a stuffed dog for a real dog) form part of the process through which a child develops abstract thought.

Vygotsky [1976] clarified the way that the transformation from concrete to abstract thought occurs. He explained that thought is separated from an object when in play, for example, a stick becomes a horse. The mechanism that causes the transition in play is that the stick 'becomes a pivot for severing the meaning of horse from a real horse' [*Vygotsky*, 1976, p. 546]. It is only in play that young children's thought is freed from real-life situational constraints.

Several researchers have demonstrated a developmental sequence from the concrete to the abstract in play. *Fein* [1975] noted that initially the child relies on an object which is prototypical; however, as the child's thinking matures, she or he is able to use a less similar object to symbolize another object in play. A somewhat similar sequence was described by *Watson and Fischer* [1977] in the progression from using the self as agent to using objects as agents. Following *Piaget* [1962], *Fenson and Ramsay* [1980] discussed this progression as a reflection of decentration, which is the process of gradually becoming less dependent on acts centered on the self. Presumably the ability to consider objects in more abstract and less centered terms, which is practised in play, would facilitate divergent problem-solving which requires the child to make a variety of free associations.

In summary, symbolic play involves using one object to signify another and is therefore an elementary form of representational thought. In play the child's thought can be severed from the concrete and moved into the abstract at an age when she or he may be otherwise incapable of abstract thought. The mechanism involved appears to be that an object (signifier) acts as a pivot or support for the symbolic representation. In play, the newly formed capacity to abstract can be practised and varied. The significance of this process for creativity presumably lies in the opportunity it provides for the child to focus beyond the obvious, to make novel associations and to engage in imaginative activity during play and subsequent divergent problem-solving.

Taken together, the theories that examine the influence of play on development suggest that play may contribute to divergent thinking by enabling the child: (a) to explore the object environment and thereby learn about it; (b) to experiment with objects and generate novel responses, and (c) to practise symbolic thinking. It remains to show whether any of these processes in play correlates with increases in creativity.

Correlates of Divergent Thinking

Having considered both the theoretical and empirical bases for the relationship between play and creativity, I now turn to an examination of the specific factors of the play experience that relate to divergent thinking. In order to understand the processes that mediate the relationship between play and creativity, I will examine research on play behaviors, individual play styles and situational factors that correlate with creative performance.

Play Behaviors that Predict Creative Performance

One strategy for clarifying the processes by which play contributes to divergent thinking is to examine the nature of children's play behavior during free play and correlate this with subsequent problem-solving performance. *Pepler* [1979] and *Pepler and Ross* [1981] conducted two studies to investigate the effects of play on divergent thinking in which these processes were examined in more detail. The children were videotaped during the three play sessions with convergent or divergent play materials. Play behaviors scored from the videotapes included behaviors relating to the form, color and representation of the play materials; investigation; construction, and symbolic play [for further details see *Pepler and Ross*, 1981]. These play behaviors were entered into a stepwise regression analysis to examine their ability to predict success on the divergent problem-solving tasks.

Despite minor inconsistencies, a general pattern of play behaviors predicting success on the divergent thinking tasks was evident. The pattern involved both investigative behaviors and behaviors in response to representation. The investigative behaviors that contributed positively to measures of divergent thinking included visual and manual investigation, and investigation of the form, dropping, and standing properties of the pieces. Through both specific and diversive investigation, the children may have learned about the properties of the pieces and their divergent uses. The children who played with the divergent materials produced significantly more of these investigative behaviors than children who played with convergent materials. Since the creativity tasks involved thinking about and reacting to the materials in as many different ways as possible, investigation of materials during play may have prepared the children for the understanding and flexibility required in the divergent thinking tasks. This class of behavior reflects the first two processes suggested by the theories relating play to divergent thinking – investigation in play and experimentation and flexibility in play.

The second class of behaviors that predicted performance on the divergent tasks included those behaviors in which the child's attention was focussed on representation, that is, what the object signified. Labelling a representation, grouping by representation, representation sounds and symbolic play are all behaviors that involve attention to the meaning of the pieces and contributed positively to predictions on the divergent tasks. Those children who during play demonstrated a shift in attention from the concrete nature of the play pieces to their more abstract meanings may have been better equipped to deal with the abstract demands of the divergent thinking tasks. Since it was primarily children in the divergent play group who grouped and played with the pieces according to representation, it was these children who were likely to be better prepared for the divergent thinking tasks. This is consistent with the third process suggested by the theories as mediating the relationship between play and creativity – play facilitates the transition from concrete to abstract thought.

In summary, the regression analyses suggested that investigative and representational play behaviors might influence performance on creativity tasks. It is important to note, however, that these analyses were correlational rather than causal. In future research, these predictive play behaviors could be manipulated and systematically examined for their individual effects on subsequent divergent problem-solving.

Individual Play Styles and Creativity

As indicated above, there have been a number of studies that demonstrate a link between play and creativity. In several of these studies particular play styles were related to creativity, suggesting that individual factors may mediate the relationship between play and creativity. These play styles appear to illustrate two of the processes postulated by the theories outlined above, namely experimentation and symbolic activity.

The process of experimentation and flexibility is suggested by the playfulness characteristics identified by *Lieberman* [1965]. She found that children who demonstrated spontaneity, joy and a sense of humor were likely to perform better on divergent thinking tasks than those who did not display these playful characteristics. Similarly, *Singer and Rummo* [1973] noted that playful, curious, and humorous children were likely to be more creative. One would assume that these children would be less constrained by the situation and more likely to explore their environment in unusual ways than children who were not playful and curious. This was also suggested by the work of *Hutt and Bhavnani* [1976], who found that boys who explored the novel toy and used it in imaginative ways were among the most creative.

The second process, that symbolic thinking in play contributes to creativity, is suggested most clearly by the work of *Dansky* [1980a]. He found that only those children whose play included make-believe elements would benefit from free play experience. On a creativity task they were able to generate more divergent uses for the objects used in play. *Pulaski* [1973] also found that children who showed a high predisposition to fantasy in free play were likely to be more imaginative in a task situation. She concluded that fantasy predisposition was the most important factor in determining the richness of fantasy production in her tasks. The importance of symbolic thinking may also be suggested by *Singer and Rummo's* [1973] study, in which they found expressiveness and communicativeness to be related to divergent thinking.

Thus, although play may provide an opportunity for all children to engage in experimentation and symbolic activity, certain children may have a predisposition for this style of play and thereby benefit more from play experience.

Situational Factors and Creativity

Having examined the characteristics of play activity and children as they relate to creativity, I will now turn to characteristics of the play situation that enhance or inhibit creativity. Research indicates that both the nonsocial (object) and social nature of the play situation relate to creativity.

The degree of structure of play materials has been found to influence creativity. *Pulaski* [1973] compared the effect of play with minimally structured play materials to play with highly structured play materials. She found that children who had previous experience with toys that did not suggest a particular play activity exhibited greater richness and variety of fantasy in a subsequent task situation. Our research [*Pepler*, 1979; *Pepler and Ross*, 1981] with convergent and divergent play materials also demonstrated this relationship – children who played with the divergent materials performed better on a measure of creativity. This difference may be accounted for by the marked differences in play behaviors with the two types of play materials. Children playing with the divergent materials engaged in more investigation, construction and symbolic play activities. The presence of a puzzle-like formboard in the convergent condition seemed to constrain play activities. Children playing with the convergent materials appeared to perceive the task demands of the materials and limited their activities to the task. Therefore, while the convergent materials provided opportunity for practising puzzle completion, they did not encourage the processes presumed to be related to creativity, namely investigation, experimentation and symbolic play. A similar observation was made by *Goldman and Chaillé* [1981], who reported that in playing with structured materials, children's activities were limited rather than flexible and experimental. Hence, they suggested that play with such structured materials would not likely foster creativity.

Additional support for the contention that highly structured materials limit creativity comes from a study by *Dreyer and Rigler* [1969], who compared children from Montessori schools to children from traditional nursery schools. They reported that children from Montessori schools, in which the materials are highly structured, were less creative than children from nursery schools. It appears that structured materials may provide such strong direction for children's activity that they inhibit the behaviors that might contribute to divergent thinking.

In addition to the influence of the structure of play materials, there is some research to suggest that social play is more conducive to creativity than solitary play. *Johnson* [1976] reported high correlations between social fantasy play and divergent thinking measures, but found no such correlations for nonsocial fantasy play. *Griffing* [1981] also reported higher correlations between sociodramatic play and imagination than between nonsociodramatic play and imagination scores. Perhaps the additional requirement to communicate and share pretense in sociodramatic play enhances symbolic thinking, which is presumed to be a mechanism in play that contributes to creativity.

Other situational factors [*Darvill, Johnson and Ershler*, this volume], such as adult intervention, may also influence the development of creativity through play. For example, there are several play training studies that demonstrate a link between fantasy play training and creativity [*Dansky*, 1980b; *Feitelson and Ross*, 1973]. In addition, the manner in which parents provide for play in the home environment has been found to relate to creativity [*Bishop and Chace*, 1971].

Clearly, there are many aspects of the child's play environment that combine to promote creative activity. Further research is required to identify more precisely those factors that provide opportunities for investigation, experimentation and symbolic activity and hence for creativity.

In summary, it would appear that the relationship between play and creativity is complex and depends on several factors. First, some characteristics of the individual, such as a playful attitude which transfers from a free-play to a task situation, may underlie the link between play and creativity. Second, certain play activities, such as experiencing novel responses or symbolic uses of objects, may be important in enhancing creativity. Finally, there may be factors of the play situation, such as unstructured materials, other children, or adults, that elicit play activities that in turn promote divergent thinking. In conducting research concerning this relationship it is imperative to recognize the complexity of the link between play and creativity and attempt to isolate the specific elements of the play experience that enhance divergent thinking.

Conclusion

There is a considerable body of research that demonstrates a link between play and creativity and suggests some of the theoretical processes underlying this relationship. There are, however, several issues that remain to be addressed, many of which stem from methodological differences among the studies. First we must determine the best measure of divergent thinking. In the studies reviewed above there is no methodological consensus: In some studies [*Johnson*, 1976] divergent thinking was measured by the number of responses, whereas in others [*Pepler*, 1979; *Pulaski*, 1973] it was measured by the originality of responses. Second, in some studies researchers have focussed on solitary play [*Pepler*, 1979] while others have centered on social play [*Johnson*, 1976] as related to divergent thinking. It is now important to systematically examine these two forms of play to identify the common or different processes that may mediate the relationship with creativity. Third, since the time lapse between the treatment (i.e., play) and the task situations varies markedly across the studies and there have been no long-term studies of the relationship between play and creativity, little is known about the durability or stability of the effect. Finally, the nature of the effect of play on divergent thinking remains unclear. On the one hand, there may be something that is transferred directly from the play to task situations. For example, a new association to an object discovered in play may be evoked in response to the divergent thinking task. On the other hand, something more general, such as a flexible response set or a playful attitude may transfer from the play to problem-solving situation. The effect of play on divergent thinking is likely dependent on a combination of these processes, but this must be delineated more clearly.

The task now facing us is to step back from the research to consider the practical implications of the presumed link between play and creativity. In order to foster the divergent thinking of preschool children, certain aspects of the play situation, such as the structure of materials and the type of play behaviors may be manipulated and stimulated for a more diverse play experience. In addition, individual differences in the predisposition for creativity should be identified, examined and fostered for their potential in helping children face the divergent problems of everyday life.

References

Berlyne, D.E.: Structure and direction in thinking (Wiley, New York 1965).

Bishop, D.W.; Chace, C.A.: Parental conceptual systems, home play environment and potential creativity in children. J. exp. Child Psychol. *12:* 318–338 (1971).

Bruner, J.: Competence in infants; in Anglin, Beyond the information given (Norton, New York 1973).

Bruner, J.: Child's play. New Scient. *62:* 126–128 (1974).

Dansky, J.L.: Make-believe: a mediator of the relationship between play and associative fluency. Child Dev. *51:* 576–579 (1980a).

Dansky, J.L.: Cognitive consequences of sociodramatic play and exploration training for economically disadvantaged preschoolers. J. Child Psychol. Psychiat. allied Disc. *20:* 47–58 (1980b).

Dansky, J.L.; Silverman, I.W.: Effects of play on associative fluency in preschool children. Devl Psychol. *9:* 38–43 (1973).

Dansky, J.L.; Silverman, I.W.: Play: a general facilitator of associative fluency. Devl Psychol. *11:* 104 (1975).
Dreyer, A.; Rigler, D.: Cognitive performance in Montessori and nursery school children. J. educ. Res. *62:* 411–416 (1969).
Fein, G.G.: A transformational analysis of pretending. Devl Psychol. *11:* 291–296 (1975).
Feitelson, W.; Ross, G.S.: The neglected factor – play. Hum. Dev. *16:* 202–223 (1973).
Fenson, L.; Ramsay, D.: Decentration and integration of the child's play in the second year. Child Dev. *51:* 171–178 (1980).
Goldman, J.; Chaillé, C.: Object use in the preschool: an under-developed resource. Biennial Meet. Soc. Res. Child Dev. 1981.
Griffing, P.: Follow-up study of sociodramatic play among black schoolage children representing two social class groups. Biennial Meet. Soc. Res. Child Dev. 1981.
Hutt, C.: Towards a taxonomy and conceptual model of play; in Hutt, Rogers, Hutt, Developmental processes in early childhood (Routledge & Kegan Paul, London, in press, 1982).
Hutt, C.; Bhavnani, R.: Predictions from play; in Bruner, Jolly, Sylva, Play – its role in development and evolution (Penguin, Middlesex 1976).
Johnson, J.E.: Relations of divergent thinking and intelligence test scores with social and nonsocial make-believe play of preschool children. Child Dev. *47:* 1200–1203 (1976).
Li, A.K.F.: Effects of play on novel responses of preschool children. Alberta J. educ. Res. *24:* 31–36 (1978).
Lieberman, J.N.: Playfulness and divergent thinking. An investigation of their relationship at the kindergarten level. J. gen. Psychol. *107:* 219–224 (1965).
Pepler, D.J.: The effects of play on convergent and divergent problem solving; Diss. University of Waterloo (unpublished, 1979).
Pepler, D.J.; Ross, H.S.: The effects of play on convergent and divergent problem solving. Child Dev. *52:* 1202–1210 (1981).
Piaget, J.: Play, dreams and imitation in childhood (Norton, New York 1962).
Pulaski, M.A.: Toys and imaginative play; in Singer, The child's world of make-believe (Academic Press, New York 1973).
Singer, D.G.; Rummo, J.: Ideational creativity and behavioral style in kindergarten aged children. Devl Psychol. *8:* 154–161 (1973).
Smilansky, S.: The effects of sociodramatic play on disadvantaged preschool children (Wiley, New York 1968).
Sutton-Smith, B.: The role of play in cognitive development. Young Children *22:* 361–370 (1967).
Sutton-Smith, B.: Novel responses to toys. Merrill-Palmer Q. *14:* 151–158 (1968).
Sutton-Smith, B.: The useless made useful: play as variability training. School Rev. *83:* 197–214 (1975).
Vygotsky, L.S.: Play and its role in the mental development of the child; in Bruner, Jolly, Sylva, Play – its role in development and evolution (Penguin, Middlesex 1976).
Watson, M.W.; Fischer, K.W.: A developmental sequence of agent use in late infancy. Child Dev. *48:* 828–836 (1977).
Weisler, A.; McCall, R.: Exploration and play. Am. Psychol. *31:* 492–508 (1976).

Contr. hum. Dev., vol. 6, pp. 79–96 (Karger, Basel 1982)

Object Play and Problem-Solving: Methodological Problems and Conceptual Promise

J.A. Cheyne

University of Waterloo, Waterloo, Ont., Canada

Although extensive and frequently spirited object manipulation may commonly be observed among a variety of birds and mammals [*Beck*, 1980], play directed toward inanimate objects has been claimed to be sufficiently frequent among primates to qualify as a specialty of the order [*Bernstein*, 1962]. If not a specialty of the order, it is clearly an outstanding characteristic of at least the anthropoid apes and human children as documented over the years [*Bruner* et al., 1976; *Groos*, 1898, 1901]. Despite more than a century of speculation about the function of such activity, only recently have empirical studies begun to document the functions of object-play in children.

Why a Functional Analysis?

It may well be argued that the problem of play is simply the result of an artificial postindustrial distinction between play and work [*Leighton and Kluckhohn*, 1947]. This is not to say that children in nonindustrialized societies do not engage in assimilative and happy interchanges with objects and people or in fantasy ideation [but see *Feitelson*, 1977]. Yet, it may be objected that these are not necessarily seen by members of all cultures as frivolous and nonfunctional activities. Many of the activities of children we would clearly label as play are, or were, viewed, by members of various societies as definite training for socially relevant roles. Indeed, from time to time, such activities are suggested and organized by adults. Moreover, family members may often fashion play objects for children in the apparent belief that they will thereby promote learning of certain social roles [*Goodman*, 1970]. Clearly that which we label as play is, in many cultures, closely integrated into everyday practical reality [*Feitelson*, 1977].

Since many nontechnological societies do not provide an abundance of toys as we know them, it has been suggested that much object play is constructive in nature [*Goodman*, 1970]. Although *Feitelson* [1977] has argued that assertions regarding the ubiquity of play are based on scant evidence, most of her arguments are relevant only to representational play and not to object play in general. Nonetheless, even if object play is universal and perceived to be functional by members of at least some cultures, it is still a valid question to ask whether object play really does promote the acquisition of general or specific skills that are either ecologically or culturally meaningful.

Some authors seem to feel that any attempt to ask functional questions of a phenomenon is tantamount to justification of the phenomenon. *Vandenberg* [1980] seems to argue in this vein by implying that those who seek a functional analysis of play by relating it to something 'important', such as problem-solving must therefore consider play inherently unimportant. Certainly, play is a delightful human attribute worthy, in its own right, of study and admiration. However, while I am somewhat sympathetic to the thrust of *Vandenberg's* [1980] argument I feel it misses the biological point of a functional analysis. Ultimately, one wishes to understand the role of animal capacities and tendencies in terms of fitness. Linking play to problem-solving is simply one small step in that direction. The role of problem-solving in determining fitness is, of course, a problem no less at issue and is indeed the subject of considerable study at many levels. On the assumption that problem-solving constitutes one plausible path through which play may impact on fitness, this review will be focused on studies that have attempted to link object play with problem-solving (i.e., the attainment of some goal via the overcoming of obstacles). Studies of the influence of play on styles of thinking (e.g., creativity) will be of less concern for this review [*Dansky and Silverman*, 1973, 1975; *Hutt and Bhavnani*, 1972] and certain tasks used by *Pepler* [1979] and *Pepler and Ross* [1981] since the tasks used do not involve problem-solving, as has been noted by several investigators [*Smith and Dutton*, 1979; *Vandenberg*, in press].

Object Play and Problem-Solving

Characterizing the nature of interactions with objects has been a perennial stumbling block for researchers. In recent years, some conceptual clarity has been achieved by a general acceptance of a distinction between exploration of and play with objects [*Hutt*, 1970; *Weisler and McCall*, 1976].

It seems to me that the exploration-play distinction is, philosophically, a very profound one. *Hutt* [1970] refers to the former as stimulus referent and to the latter as response referent. More incisive is her summary characterization of exploration as an agent posing the question: 'What can this object do?' and of play as an agent posing the question: 'What can I do with this object?' or as *Sylva* [1974] put the latter question: 'Which actions can be performed on this object?' One may also capture the spirit of this difference by paraphrasing a Shavian gem so favored by a recent United States president by saying that the exploring child sees the world as it is and asks: 'Why?'; while the playful child sees a world that never was and asks: 'Why not?' Now these are two fundamentally different ways of asking questions about the nature of the world or, more precisely, about our understanding of the world. Let me rephrase the questions slightly. Consider the question: 'What is this theory about?' and the question: 'What can I use this theory for?' The first is the traditional question of the realist who questions the truth value of theories in the literal sense. Truth is to be discovered by the explorer of the real world. The second is the Machian view that theories are not so much truthful as useful. Reality is the best creation devised by the cleverest inventor. The equation of the realist-positivist distinction with the exploration-play distinction does not, I suppose, shed any light on the relative merits of the positions but may suggest the psychological origins of the conceptual frameworks underlying the two positions. Both represent basic psychological modes of analyzing and coping with the world around us. This would not be the first instance of a philosophical dispute being based on alternate and equally valid psychological premises [*Hochberg*, 1962].

Play may thus be seen as a set or orientation that leads to the extraction from experience of instruments (tools and procedures) which can usefully be applied to problematic situations potentially far removed from the play situation. Indeed, discussions of tool use in nonhuman primates (usually chimpanzees) is generally closely associated with considerations of object play [*Bruner*, 1972; *Candland* et al., 1978; *Van Lawick-Goodall*, 1970; but see *McGrew*, 1977]. *Schiller* [1952], for instance, reports a perfect correlation between amount of object manipulation and success in tool use in a cross-age, cross-specific comparison of primates. There is also a literature suggesting that deprivation of object play opportunities leads to severely limited tool use and/or problem-solving capacity in chimpanzees [*Bernstein*, 1962; *Birch*, 1945a, b; *Jackson*, 1942; *Menzel* et al., 1970; *Schiller*, 1952]. Several of the studies used modifications of the classic stick problem described by *Hobhouse* [1901] and *Kohler* [1926]. In general the problems involve the retrieval of a lure (food) placed out of reach, the solution of which involves the use of a stick or probe which serves as an extending tool. *Kohler's* [1926] work, in particular, inspired considerable research using this paradigm. This research was rapidly extended to the investigation of the problem-solving skills of infants and young children [*Alpert*, 1928; *Brainard*, 1930; *Ling*, 1946; *Matheson*, 1931; *Menzel* et al., 1970; *Moriya*, 1937a, b; *Richardson*, 1932, 1934]. These studies, by and large, focused on the problem-solving skills per se often describing in great detail the behavior of the children in the problem situation.

Recently, the *Kohler* [1926] paradigm was reintroduced for children in a seminal study [*Sylva*, 1974, 1977; *Sylva* et al., 1976]. The focus of the study was not, however, on problem-solving but on the prior play activity with materials relevant to problem solution. Since this study is widely cited and has inspired imitators who have followed the original procedures rather closely, it deserves close scrutiny.

The task devised and employed by *Sylva* and her collaborators was very similar to the original task reported by *Kohler* [1926]. The lure (a piece of chalk) was not only out of reach but also inside a transparent latched box. The child was required to obtain the lure while remaining seated at a distance from the box. The box was so placed that the lure could be reached only by connecting two long sticks with a 'C' clamp provided, releasing the latch and then raking in the lure. The children were not, however, left entirely to their own devices. The experimenter sat near the child and provided hints when the child indicated a desire to leave or ignored the task for at least 1 min. The hints were presented in the following order:

'Have you used everything you can think of that might help you?'

'Can you think of a way that you can use the clamp to help you?'

'Can you think of a way that you can use both the clamp and the sticks to help you?'

'You could clamp the two sticks together and make a longer stick.'

'I will hold these two sticks together here. Can you clamp them tightly together with this clamp?'

In the final instance *Sylva* indicated that the child was given direct physical assistance if he or she was unable to follow directions. This basic paradigm, including the use of the specific hints has been used in a number of subsequent investigations [*Darvill*, 1981; *Smith and Dutton*, 1979; *Vandenberg*, in press].

In the *Sylva* study, prior to the presentation of the problem, children had been exposed to one of three conditions: a period of free play with the sticks and clamps, a brief demonstration of the construction of a two-stick tool using a 'C' clamp; or a very brief demonstration of the operation of a 'C' clamp. The results, by all criteria, indicated the inferiority of the third (control) group in problem-solving in comparison to the two experimental groups. Unfortunately, the poor performance of the control group in comparison to the other groups is difficult to evaluate since the children in the control group had only about 1 min of experience in the situation before being presented with the problem while the demonstrate-principle group had 2 min and the play group had 10 min of prior experience. Hence, it is difficult to attribute the superior performance of the play and demonstrate principle groups solely to the manipulated aspects of their prior experience per se since the relatively abrupt presentation of the problem task may have actively inhibited performance of the control group. Moreover, during the play period the children in the play group may have taken the opportunity to look about the room and to habituate to the novel or otherwise distracting features of the experimental situation. A control of the sort used in the *Sylva* study allows only the vaguest of conclusions regarding the nature of the advantage to the children under the play condition.

The performances of the two experimental groups were highly similar. For example, in the play group 39% of the children solved the problem without hints and in the demonstration condition 42% of the children did so, a difference of 1 subject. However, *Sylva* et al. [1976] repeatedly attempted to impute superiority to the play condition. For example, they reported that children in the play group required significantly fewer hints to solve the problem than did children in the demonstrate-principle group. However, uniquely in that paper [*Sylva* et al., 1976] a test statistic is simply presented (a Mann-Whitney U test) without an accompanying table showing the nature of the difference and making no mention of the actual number of hints required by the children or why the control group was not included in the analysis. An examination of *Sylva's* [1974, table 6] data reveals that the play, demonstrate-principle, and control groups received 74, 79 and 128 hints, respectively. Clearly inclusion of the data from the control group in any analysis reveals the trivial magnitude of the difference between the play and demonstrate-principle groups. In any case, as we shall see, the use of hints represents a serious flaw in the procedure employed by *Sylva*, and its use as a dependent variable is particularly problematic.

Sylva et al. [1976] described the children in the play group as more active during the problem-solving phase and more organized in their approach to solving the problem than the children in the demonstrate-principle group. The evidence presented in support of this conclusion consists of apparent differences between the two groups in the number and variety of goal-directed responses in the problem-solving situation. However, later in the report, we are informed that there were more immediate solvers in the demonstrate-principle group than in the play group. This is not surprising since the children in the demonstrate-principle group had just been shown the principle. It does mean, however, that more of the children under the demonstrate-principle condition than under the play condition were precluded from showing a number of strategies because they solved the problem on one of their initial attempts. Moreover, it seems a reasonable assumption that, in terms of problem-solving, the brighter children in the demonstrate-principle group would have benefited from the demonstration and would have been among the immediate problem solvers. The very children under the demonstrate-principle condition who were most likely to have demonstrated orderliness in their problem-solving attempts have thus selectively removed themselves from inclusion in the sample that contributed to the measure of orderliness. Thus, all the measures of number, quality and orderliness of problem-solving attempts reduce to a restatement of the fact that children in the demonstrate-principle group who were able to solve the problem did so more directly than children in the play group.

A further methodological concern arises from the use of a yoked control design in *Sylva's* second experiment. *Sylva* used two yoked control groups. Under one condition a child watched an adult make the same configurations as a child under the play condition had made. Under another condition, a child was guided by an adult as he or she made the same configurations as a child under the play condition had made. Thus, each child under the play condition had two yoked control 'partners'. *Sylva* [1974] saw this as a test for configurational richness. Why she did so is not clear since the yoked control children experienced the same configurations as the play children and hence were exposed to the same specific features of the configurations, the same operations involved in their construction, the same stages of development of the constructions and had the same opportunity to extract specific principles from these experiences. To conclude that the yoked control children were exposed to configurational richness in an any less confounded sense than the play children is quite unjustified. The fact that, for the number of hints required for problem-solving, there were significant correlations between the play children and both of their yoked control partners simply provides evidence that *something*, quite unspecified, about the configurations or their formation made a difference in the number of hints given in the problem situation. There is, however, a more serious problem resulting from the use of yoked control procedures in this paradigm.

Before drawing conclusions from studies employing yoking strategies one would do well to consider *Church's* [1964] critique of yoked control designs. Yoked control designs will be biased (usually negatively) when there is systematic variability in the response of the subjects to the treatment which is the basis for the yoking. Now this is true almost by definition in the case of play. *Sylva* [1974, pp. 84, 85] was very sensitive to this argument and imagined the following troubling scenario: 'Suppose that the very bright children were enormously benefited by watching complex constructions whereas duller children do not so profit. Now suppose that being exposed to a barren configuration affected both bright and dull children equally.' If this were true then the yoking would be biased since the brighter children were handicapped by receiving the poorer configurations while the dulle children were not helped by observing the richer configurations. This would, of course, lower the over-all level of performance of the yoked control subjects making the experimental group look spuriously proficient. *Sylva* [1974] dismissed this possibility, arguing that although a bright child might have been hindered by exposure to an especially impoverished configuration, a dull child might have been helped as much by an especially rich one. This is, of course, simply the logical fallacy of 'denying the antecedent' and is, moreover, contrary to anything one would expect from differences in intelligence. Furthermore, if one assumes that, in the *Sylva* [1974] study, the proportion of solvers in the play condition is a reasonable estimate of the proportion of competent children in the population under study and that they produce the appropriate number of configurations then one can predict the expected proportion of solvers in the yoked control group to be the square of the proportion of solvers in the play group. The proportion of children in the play group who solved the problem without hints was 0.39 or 14/36. Thus, the predicted proportion based on this logic is 0.152 or 6/36. The obtained proportion for each of the two yoked control groups is 0.167 and 0.194 or 6/36 and 7/36. I claim a remarkably close fit and conclude that the yoked control subjects given the appropriate configurations do as well as the play children who produced them spontaneously.

The final and, because it applies with equal or greater force to subsequent research, potentially most serious flaw in the *Sylva* design concerns the failure to use double-blind procedures. Recently, the ape-language research has come under rather spirited attack on the issue of the Clever Hans effect [*Sebeok and Sebeok*, 1980]. Clever Hans was one of a long line of justly famous animals of allegedly prodigious intellectual powers. Clever Hans was a horse with especial facility in mathematics. That Hans majored in math is not surprising given that his teacher was a retired mathematics teacher, Mr. von Osten. It is interesting, though undoubtedly futile, to speculate about whether it was Mr. von Osten's success with his human pupils, or lack of it, that drove him to tutor his horse. Hans did have other, nonmathematcal, abilities, not usually possessed by horses, including, from time to tiime flashes of psychic power. Clever Hans is among the most famous of the clever animals partly because of the painstaking and ingenious research of the psychologist *Pfungst* who demonstrated that the questioners themselves unwittingly provided Hans with answers, or rather, with cues that permitted him to respond as though he knew the answers. Hans certainly did possess remarkable perceptual acuity and showed a lot of horse sense in the way he responded to the odd behaviors of his questioners. Of mathematics, however, knew neither jot nor tittle and probably knew little Latin and less Greek. Mr. von Osten, it is interesting to note, never did accept the evidence of *Pfungst* and continued to believe in the abilities of Hans. One does worry about all the other pupils of Mr. von Osten.

The subtlety and power of the Clever Hans effect is indeed sobering [*Pfungst*, 1911]. The ability of animals including humans of all ages to garner nonverbal cues and to use them to direct and guide their behavior in rather subtle ways should not be disregarded or underestimated in play studies. In these studies the impact of interpersonal factors is undeniable. Of particular concern is the role of the experimenter in providing hints to children based on criteria that are somewhat subject to interpretation. Indeed, in *Sylva's* study the experimenter was not merely interacting with the child but was, in fact, instructing the child in task specifics. This would seem to put a remarkable strain on the experimenter's objectivity. My concern for this grows, in part, from a finding in some pilot work in which an attempt was being made to replicate *Sylva's* findings. We were attempting to determine, in addition, correlations between specific behaviors during play and problem-solving proficiency. One of the strongest correlations to emerge from the analysis was between task proficiency and the amount of visual regard of the experimenter by the child during the problem-solving phase of the study. One might offer several hypotheses as to why this should be so. One of the more compelling and troubling is the Clever Hans hypothesis.

The danger of the Clever Hans effect, though not ignored, has not been addressed with sufficient vigour in research on play and problem-solving. If the Clever Hans effect has capitalized on experimenter bias then we are undone. *Sylva* did not use double-blind procedures and presents some plausible reasons for not doing so. She did attempt to control for experimenter bias by running a small number of subjects with naive experimenters. However, because of extremely small numbers (around 3 per cell) the results are ambiguous. Moreover, we do not know whether the naive observer was alone with the child or whether the original experimenter was also present. *Sylva*, and most other researchers have been concerned more with experimenter bias in recording than with direct biasing of the child's behavior by the experimenter. For example, *Pepler* [personal communication; see also *Pepler*, 1979; *Pepler and Ross*, 1981] reported that she used a naive observer to control for bias in recording, although the experimenter remained in the room with the child and the observer. Thus, although recording bias was controlled for, the Clever Hans effect was not. *Vandenberg* [in press] seems, like *Pepler* to have controlled for bias in recording but not for the Clever Hans effect. It should be noted, however, that *Vandenberg* [in press] reported that the observer sat behind the child during the play phase. It is not clear where the experimenter sat when the second experimenter entered the room. The second experimenter is described, however, only as recording. Presumably, it was the original experimenter who was interacting with the child, giving hints, etc. *Smith and Dutton* [1979] seem not to have considered or controlled for experimenter or observer bias at all. It is interesting to note, in passing, that *Smith and Dutton* [1979] have obtained the most clear-cut and powerful effects of play on problem-solving ability.

Now it may be, as in language acquisition, that the Clever Hans effect is an integral part of the learning process. This is not uninteresting. However, it is important to know just what the facts are. Now I wish to underline that I do not think that the Clever Hans hypothesis, if correct, impugns the importance of the current research. It may simply be that, as in the original case of Clever Hans, the phenomenon, though interesting, is not what it seems. One is almost tempted to say that it is a horse of a different color.

Vandenberg [in press] repeated *Sylva's* study using a similar lure-retrieval problem and found that the play group performed better than a nonplay control group using a measure of task proficiency based on hints. He failed, however, to obtain such an effect when he used a somewhat different task. There were, however, a number of differences in the procedures used in the two studies. In *Vandenberg's* study, children in the play group were allowed 10 min of play with relevant materials as in *Sylva's* study. However, *Vandenberg* attempted to equate the groups for experience with the materials by having control children answer questions about the physical and comparative aspects of the materials for a 10-min period. He also endeavored to provide some familiarity with the setting prior to treatment by allowing all children a period of 10 min to play in the setting with warm-up materials (Lego blocks). Perhaps the choice of object play as a warm-up activity, especially with such similar materials, attenuated the difference between play and nonplay groups. Nevertheless, *Vandenberg* did obtain a play effect on the task most like *Sylva's*. *Vandenberg's* failure to find an effect on the second task probably resulted from a combination of the very large age range he used, 4–10 years, and the fact that the means for older children under both conditions were very near asymptote (10.2 and 10.4 of a possible 11 points in the second task). Thus, attempts to draw conclusions from this task difference [*Pepler and Ross*, 1981; *Vandenberg*, in press] would seem unwarranted.

Smith and Dutton [1979] followed up *Sylva's* work with the addition of a simple extension (literally!) of the lure retrieval problem. They closely replicated *Sylva's* procedures obtaining highly similar results. When children had successfully solved the lure retrieval problem with a double-stick construction, they were presented with the problem again. However, on the second occasion the lure was placed still further away, requiring a three-stick construction for solution. *Smith and Dutton* [1979] suggested that this latter problem requires an 'innovative' solution. Indeed, it seems that this was a particularly 'sticky' problem and did present additional difficulties for the preschool children, for they took as long or longer to solve the second problem under training and control conditions. The children under the play condition, on the other hand, achieved the innovative solution more rapidly than they did their first solution. Either they were able both to use their experience in the first problem and to elaborate upon that experience or something about the play experience otherwise prepared them for problems requiring more elaborate solutions. *Smith and Dutton* [1979] found this to be true for solution time as well as for number of hints given. This is a very exciting finding and deserves scrutiny and replication. Unfortunately, although the use of solution time as well as number of hints given is a definite strength, their study contains many of the same methodological flaws as *Sylva's* (e.g., the extensive use of hints and the complete failure to control for experimenter bias or the Clever Hans effect). A particular weakness of this study lies in the fact that apparently only one experimenter was employed, who demonstrated, observed, gave hints and recorded all dependent variables. Moreover, no reliability data are given for any of the dependent variables of the study. The problem of bias induced by hints is somewhat mitigated by the finding that, for the second problem, there were more children under the play condition who required hints than under the other conditions. Nonetheless, it would be reassuring to see this study repeated with more adequate control procedures.

There is one limitation of *Sylva's* study that *Smith and Dutton's* study overcame, to a degree. In *Sylva's* study the demonstrate-principle and two of the control groups were at a considerable disadvantage inasmuch as they had no opportunity to handle the materials at all. *Smith and Dutton* [1979] gave all children a 2-min period in which they were permitted to manipulate the materials. The authors suggested that this manipulation may have served, at least partially, to equate the groups on exploration. Had all children been given a longer period of familiarization with the setting, as in the *Vandenberg's* [in press] study, experience with the setting and with the specific materials would have more nearly equated the groups on nonplay factors.

As indicated previously, *Smith and Dutton* [1979] referred to the solution of the second problem as requiring innovation or flexible thinking and suggest that the play group excelled in this aspect of problem-solving. This does not necessarily follow, however. For the training and control groups, the joining of three sticks was clearly an innovation since they had not been shown or otherwise exposed to such a configuration. On the other hand, the children in the play group may well have made three-stick constructions in play. Hence, for these children the second problem may have required no more or less innovation than the first problem. Unfortunately, *Smith and Dutton* [1979] did not report any measures of play construction that might have shed light on this issue. Thus, their study does not provide evidence that play leads to greater innovation or flexibility in problem-solving which the authors take as their major conclusion [*Smith and Dutton*, 1979, p. 335].

Rubin et al. [in press] also have difficulty with *Smith and Dutton's* concept of innovation since they feel the initial discovery of the principle of extension requires more innovation than the mere iterative use of the same principle (with a third stick). This problem may arise from a misunderstanding of *Smith and Dutton's* meaning of innovation. These investigators appear to have been focusing on the demonstrate-principle condition and saw solution of the two-stick problem as a simple application of the principle as demonstrated, whereas the solution of the three-stick problem required the children to go beyond literal imitation. However, as has been pointed out, since *Smith and Dutton* [1979] did not analyze constructions made by the children we have no idea whether or not this was true of children in the play group. Given this error on the part of *Smith and Dutton*, the question raised by *Rubin* et al. [in press] concerning which task required the more innovative solution for the play group remains to be answered.

Pepler [1979] and *Pepler and Ross* [1981] expanded somewhat on the issue of the function of play by considering both problem-solving and divergent thinking. They used a variety of problem-solving tasks that were quite different from the lure-retrieval problem used in the previous research. *Pepler* also employed a number of nonplay control groups with which to compare the play group. Children in the play groups were allowed three 10-min play sessions with a variety of blocks in animate and inanimate shapes. In one control group, the children spent an equivalent amount of time doing puzzles (using the same materials). In the first experiment, children in two other groups observed either puzzle-solving or play-like manipulation of the materials by the experimenter. In the second study, the latter two groups were replaced by a more conventional control group that had no exposure to the materials but spent an equivalent period of time reading books with the experimenter. In the first experiment, *Pepler* [1979] found the play groups to be superior to the control groups on one of two tests of divergent thinking but not on any of her three problem-solving tests. In the second experiment, the play group was again found to be superior on a divergent thinking task, in this case one directly modified from *Dansky and Silverman* [1973]. Again, however, no effects were found for measures of problem-solving. Given *Pepler's* [1979] failure to find any effects of play on problem-solving it seems an important task for researchers to begin to investigate a wider array of problems than those involving tool construction for lure retrieval.

The Question: 'How?'

Unlike *Smith and Dutton* [1979], most researchers in the field have attempted to observe and record the behaviors of the children during the play session. Given that one does find evidence that play impacts on problem-solving proficiency one would like to attempt to determine how this efficacy is achieved. A first step toward this latter goal is to look for components of play that correlate with problem-solving performance.

At least as far back as *Groos* [1898, 1901], it has been speculated that one of the potential functions of play is to provide the organism with specific skills for a variety of life tasks. Both *Birch* [1945b] and *Schiller* [1952] provide strong evidence that fairly specific skills and principles, with regard to sticks and other objects as tools, are learned in unconstrained, playful object manipulation. Recently, evidence from research with children has accumulated to suggest that task-specific skills may be built up in the context of object play [*Cheyne and Rubin*, 1981; *Darvill*, 1981; *Pepler and Ross*, 1981; *Vandenberg*, in press]. In particular, *Darvill* [1981] has provided experimental evidence that play in which learning and practice of task-specific skills and principles are precluded degrades the efficacy of play in facilitating problem-solving. While it now appears clear that play does promote the learning of specific skills and principles, it remains to be clarified in what manner and at what levels these skills and principles are learned. The implications of the answers to these questions extend beyond theories of play and will be discussed briefly in the following and final section.

Sylva made several attempts to relate components of play to task performance. This was done, indirectly, when *Sylva* et al. [1976] concluded, from the correlation between task scores of children in the play group and their yoke mates, that configurational richness affects task performance. *Vandenberg* [1980] criticized this conclusion since there was no assessment of, or attempt to define, configurational richness in the report by *Sylva* et al. [1976]. However, *Sylva* [1974] did precisely define configurational richness and directly related it to task performance. She defined poor configurations as involving less than five single clampings and 'rich' configurations as those involving more than four single clampings or at least one double-stick clamping. She found that children in the play group who made 'rich' configurations were significantly more likely to be spontaneous solvers (11 of 15 subjects) than children who made 'poor' configurations (3 of 21) subjects. She reported that this relation also held for children under the yoked control conditions but not as powerfully as for the children under the play condition. Although *Vandenberg* [in press] was unable to replicate this finding, more recent work found a significant correlation between configurational richness and solution time [*Cheyne and Rubin*, 1981]. This relation was obtained for a measure very similar to that used by *Sylva* [1974]. Evidence was less strong for a measure similar to that used by *Vandenberg* [in press]. Once again, however, these are merely correlational findings which may simply mean that play is a potential means of assessing problem-solving ability. What is needed now is an experimental study in which configurational richness is manipulated. This might be a study of the sort conducted by *Darvill* [1981] who manipulated the performance or nonperformance of task specifics by altering the characteristics of the materials.

Problem-Solving: Insight as Recollection

As noted earlier in this paper, the primary concern of *Kohler* [1926] and many of those early investigators who applied his paradigm to young children was the investigation of problem-solving. Thus, these investigators tended to focus on, and describe in great detail, the behavior of the children in the problem situation to the relative exclusion of a consideration of the child's prior experience with the materials in nonproblematic situations. More recent research has, in contrast, tended to focus on the nonproblematic, playful object manipulation and make only summary observations of problem-solving effectiveness. Some research, notably that of *Birch* [1945a] and *Schiller* [1952, 1957] with chimpanzees and of *Pepler* [1979] and *Pepler and Ross* [1981] with children, has been less one-sided, although in the cases of *Birch* and *Schiller* it is often difficult to distinguish play and problem-solving contexts from their descriptions.

That the remaining research has been relatively one-sided is unfortunate because the functional model of play that one arrives at will have implications for models of problem-solving. It seems to me, for example, that *Schiller's* interpretation of the consequences of play leads to an implicit model of problem-solving (only partly explicated by *Schiller*). According to this author, the performance of a principle emerged in play at an earlier age than in the problem situation. Thus, the youngest animal to connect the sticks in play was 6-year-old while the youngest to do so in the problem context was 8. Moreover, among *Schiller's* animals the problem was never solved by animals who had not made the necessary connection in play. He concluded from this that, to be used for problem-solving 'the pattern must be readily available before it can emerge, and it is not the pressure of the need that makes it emerge, but, on the contrary, such a pressure represses, if it is not highly available' [*Schiller*, 1957, p. 272]. This, of course, sounds reminiscent of the classic *Yerkes-Dodson* [1908] law. Most importantly, however, *Schiller* [1957, p. 277] also reported that simple discovery was not sufficient for implementation in problem contexts and alluded to the necessity of consolidation through repetition. 'My Chimpanzees learned (the principle of joining sticks) rapidly . . . but they played a lot with the double stick before incorporating it into the problem situation . . . Repetition condenses the chain, to a unified skill pattern.' Thus, both discovery and subsequent assimilation in play are seen to be important precursors of problem-solving. More specifically, using a distinction similar to that of *Tulving and Pearlstone* [1966] one may suggest that discovery makes the principle available but assimilative activity makes it accessible. Given *Schiller's* [1952] premise that the principle must be learned in play, problem-solving becomes a process of accessing principles and perceiving them as solutions to problems at hand. Problem-solving may thus be understood as being little more than cued retrieval of information – a memory problem – the problem itself being a rather ambiguous cue. Perhaps the great advantage of play is that it opens up a number of channels of access to principles and action.

Birch's [1945a, p. 383] interpretations, on the other hand, would seem to imply that the effect of play is to better prepare the individual to generate principles during problem solving. 'In insightful problem solving, in contrast with trial and error solution, previous experience provides the materials out of which an adequate pattern of response may be fabricated rather than the stereotyped problem-solving response itself.' Thus, play may provide the opportunity for the acquisition of components, but the problem solver must 'recall and reorganize in new patterns of response previously learned, *but not contiguously learned* items of experience' [*Birch*, 1945a, p. 381, italics in original].

There have been two recent attempts to resolve the *Birch* and *Schiller* differences [*Cheyne and Rubin*, 1981; *Vandenberg*, in press]. The weight of evidence seems, at present, to favour *Schiller's* position. That is, the learning of the components (joining sticks) which must be integrated (joining long sticks to form a longer extending tool) to solve a lure-retrieval problem aids little in problem-solving whereas when the integration of the components in conformity with the principle of extension occurs in play, problem-solving is significantly enhanced [*Cheyne and Rubin*, 1981]. In any case, it would be wise to heed *Scandura's* [1977, p. 268] warning that 'it would be dangerous to assume that the differences between rule derivation and rule retrieval can be safely ignored'. Understanding the function(s) of play involves understanding the nature of play and the nature of the activities which play is hypothesized to effect.

We have barely begun to investigate the functions of play, but we now have at least a glimpse of where some answers may lie. Through a process of careful description, imaginative experimentation, and playful modelling of process, we are beginning to understand and may potentially optimize the child's understanding of the world that is, and of worlds that might be.

References

Alpert, A.: The solving of problem situations by preschool children. Teach. Coll. Contr. Educ., No. 323 (1928).

Beck, B.B.: Animal tool behavior: the use and manufacture of tools by animals (Garland, New York 1980).

Bernstein, I.S.: Response to nesting materials of wild born and captive born chimpanzees. Anim. Behav. *10:* 1–6 (1962).

Birch, H.G.: The role of motivational factors in insightful problem solving. J. comp. Psychol. *38:* 295–317 (1945a).

Birch, H.G.: The relation of previous experience to insightful problem solving. J. comp. Psychol. *38:* 267–283 (1945b).

Brainard, P.P.: The mentality of the child compared with that of the apes. J. genet. Psychol. *37:* 268–293 (1930).

Bruner, J.: The nature and uses of immaturity. Am. Psychol. *27:* 687–708 (1972).

Bruner, J.; Jolly, A.; Sylva, K.: Play: its role in development and evolution (Penguin, Middlesex 1976).

Candland, D.K.; French, J.A.; Johnson, C.N.: Object-play: test of a categorization model by the genesis of object-play in *Macaca fuscata;* in Smith, Social play in primates (Academic Press, New York 1978).

Cheyne, J.A.; Rubin, K.H.: Playful precursors of problem solving in preschoolers. Biennial Meet. Soc. for Res. in Child Dev., Boston 1981.

Church, R.M.: Systematic effect of random error in the yoked control design. Psychol. Bull. *62:* 122–131 (1964).

Dansky, J.L.; Silverman, I.W.: Effects of play on associative fluency in preschool children. Devl Psychol. *9:* 38–43 (1973).

Dansky, J.L.; Silverman, I.W.: Play: a general facilitator of associative fluency. Devl Psychol. *11:* 104 (1975).

Darvill, D.: Effect of play with relevant and non-relevant materials on problem solving; unpubl. MA thesis Waterloo (1981).

Feitelson, D.: Cross-cultural studies of representational play; in Tizard, Harvey, Biology of play (Heinemann, London 1977).

Goodman, M.E.: The culture of childhood: child's-eye views of society and culture (Teach. Coll. Press, Columbia University, New York 1970).

Groos, K.: The play of animals (Appleton, New York 1898).

Groos, K.: The play of man (Appleton, New York 1901).

Hobhouse, L.T.: Mind in evolution (MacMillan, London 1901).

Hochberg, J.E.: Nativism and empiricism in perception; in Postman, Psychology in the making: histories of selected research problems (Knopf, New York 1962).

Hutt, C.: Specific and diversive exploration; in Reese, Lipsitt, Advances in child development and behavior, vol. 5 (Academic Press, New York 1970).

Hutt, C.; Bhavnani, R.: Predictions from play. Nature, Lond. *237:* (1972).

Jackson, T.A.: Use of the stick as a tool by young chimpanzees. J. comp. Psychol. *34:* 223–235 (1942).

Kohler, W.: The mentality of apes (Harcourt, New York 1926).

Leighton, D.; Kluckhohn, C.: Children of the people (Harvard University Press, Cambridge 1947).

Ling, B.C.: The solving of problem-situations by the preschool child. J. genet. Psychol. *68:* 3–28 (1946).

Matheson, E.: A study of problem solving behavior in preschool children. Child Dev. *2:* 242–262 (1931).

McGrew, W.C.: Socialization and object manipulation of wild chimpanzees; in Chevalier-Skolnikoff, Poirier, Primate bio-social development: biological, social and ecological determinants (Garland, New York 1977).

Menzel, E.W.; Davenport, R.K.; Roger, C.M.: The development of tool using in wild-born and restriction-reared chimpanzees. Folia primatol. *17:* 273–283 (1970).

Moriya, M.: An observation of problem-solving behavior in preschool children. I. Application of the principle of the lever. Jap. J. exp. Psychol. *4:* 63–81 (1937a).

Moriya, M.: An observation on problem-solving behavior in preschool children. II. Application of the principle of the lever (continued). Jap. J. exp. Psychol. *4:* 147–160 (1937b).

Pepler, D.J.: The effects of play on convergent and divergent problem solving; unpubl. diss. Waterloo (1979).

Pepler, D.J.; Ross, H.S.: The effects of play on convergent and divergent problem solving. Child Dev. *52:* 1202–1210 (1981).

Pfungst, O.: Clever Hans: a contribution to experimental animal and human psychology (Holt, New York 1911).

Richardson, H.M.: The growth of adaptive behavior in infants: an experimental study of seven age levels. Genet. Psychol. Monogr. *12:* 195–359 (1932).

Richardson, H.M.: The adaptive behavior of infants in the utilization of the lever as a tool: a developmental and experimental study. J. genet. Psychol. *44:* 352–377 (1934).

Rubin, K.H.; Fein, G.G.; Vandenberg, B.: Play; in Hetherington, Handbook of child psychology, vol. 3, Social development (Wiley, New York, in press).

Scandura, J.M.: Problem solving: a structural/process approach with instructional implications (Academic Press, New York 1977).

Schiller, P.H.: Innate constituents of complex responses in primates. Psychol. Rev. *59:* 177–191 (1952).

Schiller, P.H.: Innate motor action as a basis of learning; in Schiller, Instinctive behavior (International Universities Press, New York 1957).

Sebeok, T.A.; Sebeok, P.J.: Speaking of apes: a critical anthology of two-way communication with man (Plenum, New York 1980).

Smith, P.K.; Dutton, S.: Play and training in direct and innovative problem solving. Child Dev. *50:* 830–836 (1979).

Sylva, K.: The relationship between play and problem-solving in children 3–5 years old; unpubl. diss. Harvard University, Cambridge (1974).

Sylva, K.: Play and learning; in Tizard, Harvey, Biology of play (Heinemann, London 1977).

Sylva, K.; Bruner, J.; Genova, P.: The role of play in the problem solving of children 3–5 years of age; in Bruner, Jolly, Sylva, Play: its role in development and evolution (Penguin, Middlesex 1976).

Tulving, E.; Pearlstone, Z.: Availability versus accessibility of information in memory for words. J. verb. Learn. verb. Behav. *5:* 381–391 (1966).

Vandenberg, B.: Play: a causal agent in problem solving? Am. Psychol. Ass. Meet., Montreal 1980.

Vandenberg, B.: The role of play in the development of insightful tool-using strategies. Merrill-Palmer Q. (in press).

Van Lawick-Goodall, J.: Tool-using in primates and other vertebrates; in Lehrman, Hinde, Shaw, Advances in the study of behavior, vol. 1, pp. 195–249 (Academic Press, New York 1970).

Weisler, A.; McCall, R.: Exploration and play. Am. Psychol. *31:* 492–508 (1976).

Yerkes, R.M.; Dodson, J.D.: The relation of the strength of the stimulus to the rapidity of habit-formation. J. comp. Neurol. Psychol. *18:* 459–482 (1908).

Contr. hum. Dev., vol. 6, pp. 97–113 (Karger, Basel 1982)

Pretend-Play Training in Childhood: A Review and Critique

Eli Saltz, Jane Brodie[1]

Wayne State University, Detroit, Mich., USA

Does 'pretend play' influence cognitive development in young children? The very question seems to arouse strong emotions in many. On the one hand, there are those for whom the notion of 'play' seems to have an almost mystic significance for development, second only to breast-feeding or mother-love. To others, the notion is treated like an attempt to invoke supernatural causation, and it arouses the type of outraged reactions evoked by words like 'Rorschach' 40 years ago.

Recent research has examined the issue by studying the effects of training children to engage in various types of pretend play. Experimenters have reported that such training has facilitated a diverse set of cognitive abilities including vocabulary and general IQ changes, problem-solving, divergent thinking, perspective taking, and impulse control. However, recently these studies have been criticized by some as poorly controlled [*Smith and Syddall*, 1978]. The critics have not necessarily challenged the findings of these studies; the criticism centers around the contention that alternative explanations for the results are possible. In the present chapter we have attempted to evaluate both the research studies and the criticisms of these studies.

Theoretical Bases for the Effects of Pretend Play

To evaluate such research we must know (a) the basic hypotheses being tested by an experiment, and (b) some of the reasonable alternatives that

[1] The writers wish to express their gratitude to the Spencer Foundation for its support in making this paper possible.

must be eliminated by appropriate control conditions. Two aspects of pretend play have been most often hypothesized as critical to cognitive development: representational activities, and role-playing. Representations refer to activities in which children pretend that something (e.g., a stick) is something else (e.g., a horse or a gun). In role-playing, children pretend that they are someone else (e.g., mother, the grocer, superman, etc.).

Vygotsky [1967] is illustrative of the theorists who focused on representational activities, in play, as an important factor in cognitive development. He noted that young children tend to be very concrete, and have difficulty using language to represent situations that are inconsistent with ongoing environmental stimuli (e.g., 2-year-olds refused to imitate a sentence stating that it is snowing unless it was indeed snowing at the time). *Vygotsky* [1967] observed that in pretend play, children begin to use language in nonliteral ways, such as pretending to ride a stick and calling the stick a horse. Here play permitted breaking the concrete relationship between the *word* 'horse' and a specific object in the world, the flesh and blood horse. Through play, the children were seen as starting on the long road to the development of representational thought, by permitting the stick to 'steal' the horse's name.

It follows from theories like *Vygotsky's* [1967] that pretend play should foster ability to think in more representational modes. This general point of view led later researchers to hypothesize that training children to engage in pretend play should facilitate the abilities of these children on a number of tasks, such as: (a) language development, since acquisition of both vocabulary and the rules of grammar appear to rely on inferential reasoning from use of language in context; (b) many of the IQ subtests, which appear to measure problem-solving skills of representation and inference; (c) divergent thinking (e.g., the *Uses* test) which appears to require ability to go beyond the concrete, immediate associations to objects; (d) impulse control, which involves the use of internalized cues in order to break the hold exercised over behavior by the immediate, concrete stimuli of the external world.

Role-playing is the second major variable that has concerned researchers in the area of pretend play. It is well documented that children have difficulties understanding the points of view of others [*Piaget*, 1932]. Theorists like *Mead* [1932] have suggested that pretend play may be a factor in the development of such understanding. In pretend play children often take the roles of others; such changes in perspective could serve as a basis for their understanding the emotions and reactions of others.

Criteria for Evaluating Pretend-Play Studies

Based on the rationale discussed above, experiments have been designed using pretend play as a means for generating both representational and role-taking activities. Results of many such experiments indicate that training children to engage in pretend play leads to superior performance on various intellectual and perspective-taking tasks, compared to children not so trained. In evaluating such experiments, the first issue becomes, did the experiments adequately control for alternative hypotheses concerning the superior performance of the children who engaged in pretend play? To answer this question, we must first decide on the most reasonable alternative hypotheses.

In training studies, there is one ubiquitous 'alternative hypothesis', a variable that is capable of improving performance across a wide range of tasks which involve quite diverse underlying abilities: increased rapport between the experimenter and the children. Even if a training technique had no effect on vocabulary development, etc. it might appear to have an effect if the trained children felt comfortable enough with the experimenter to answer his or her questions, while the control, nontrained children were shy in the presence of an unfamiliar experimenter. This factor is a potential problem in a number of the experiments that we shall examine.

For the most part, other alternative hypotheses are viable only for restricted types of outcome variables, or restricted types of training. For example, amount of verbal interaction, per se, between experimenter and children might facilitate certain language variables, like vocabulary or grammatical usage; however, it is unclear how this could influence other behaviors, like perspective-taking, unless the verbal interaction was somehow specifically concerned with perspective-taking issues. While verbal interaction has been proposed by several writers [*Smith and Syddall*, 1978; *Rubin*, 1980] as a catch-all explanation for all manner of behavior changes, the rationale for such explanations has not always been spelled out. However, as shall be seen, the data from the pretend-play training studies are too complex to support the contention that some single contaminating variable is producing all the different effects that have been found.

A second type of criterion for evaluating experiments is the reasonableness of the obtained results, given our knowledge of developmental processes. This is a potentially dangerous criterion, since it could permit ignorance and bias to lead us to reject basically sound data. On the other hand, our background of knowledge can at the very least indicate that certain types of effects must be examined very carefully before we accept them. At this point, the writers are primarily concerned with those experiments which have reported sizeable changes in relatively abstract, general abilities after only a handful of training sessions. Specific skills (e.g., learning to tie shoelaces) can be learned in few trials by appropriately developed children; even here, the training must be specific to the skill. It is more difficult to believe that two or three training sessions in pretend play could improve general representational ability so markedly that children would show general improvement in vocabulary, divergent thinking, conservation ability, and so forth. Yet, how few sessions are too few?

Major Types of Pretend Play in Training Studies

Before considering specific experiments, let us examine some types of pretend-play activities on which children have been trained, since they have different characteristics, and might be expected to lead to somewhat different outcomes.

Sociodramatic Play. We owe this term, as well as the first large-scale training experiment, to *Smilansky* [1968]. In general, the training consisted of introducing themes with which the children had previous experience, like going to the doctor, or a trip to the grocery, and encouraging the children to enact these experiences. Training was informal and consisted of intervention by the experimenter to enrich and prolong the enactment (e.g., the experimenter might ask questions like, 'How is your baby today?' in order to enrich a doctor sequence). Toys were often provided to serve as props for the enactment. In the most effective of the conditions, as described by *Smilansky*, such enactments were preceded by field trips which would serve as the bases for the enactment (e.g., a trip to a fire station, which was later reenacted).

What are the characteristics of such sociodramatic play? The play is realistic; it centers on the children's actual experiences. It involves role-taking and social interaction between children. And it involves both social representation and object representation. The social representation occurs when the children react to each other in terms of the roles that they are playing, not in terms of their actual physical and social characteristics. The object representation occurs when the children pretend that one object is really another (e.g., pretend that a doll is a baby).

Thematic Fantasy Play. Most extensively explored by *Saltz* et al. [1977], this type of pretend play involves reading fairy tales to children, then having the children reenact the stories. Reenactments were required to follow the original story line, though of course the children were not expected to memorize dialogue. Thematic fantasy play differs from sociodramatic play in several ways. First, it is less focused on the children's actual experiences than is sociodramatic play. Second, thematic fantasy play is more likely to have a strong plot, an internal, logical, dramatic structure to the course of events; sociodramatic play is usually unplotted, with little dramatic action and little necessary order to the sequence of events. Thematic fantasy play and sociodramatic play are similar, on the other hand, in that both involve role play, social interaction between children, and both social and object representation.

Story Discussion. This training procedure was studied by a number of investigators, including *Smilansky* [1968] and *Saltz* et al. [1977]. As in thematic fantasy play, children hear fairy tales in a group situation. However, instead of enacting the stories, the children discuss them, are asked questions about events and about motivation of the characters (e.g., 'Why did the wolf want to get to Red Ridinghood's grandmother's house before Red Ridinghood got there?'). Here we have verbalizations about play in a social situation, but without the physical play occurring. As in thematic fantasy play, the content is remote from the children's experiences. Also, the strong plot is present with its logical, dramatic structure and ordering of events. However, unlike sociodramatic or thematic fantasy play, while some role-taking may occur, via identification with the main characters, it is not systematic or overt. In the absence of representational responses to objects, or to the roles being played by other children, the burden of meaning is carried by language per se, a much more abstract form of representation.

Note that many other forms of pretend play can be observed in young children. These other forms have not yet been systematically examined in the context of the effects of training for pretend play.

Evaluation of Research

In examining the specific studies that have investigated the relationships between training for pretend play and various cognitive functions, we shall, for convenience, arbitrarily distinguish between three types of cognitive functioning, (a) 'intellectual' functions, (b) social perspective taking, and (c) impulse control.

'Intellectual' Functions

The intellectual functions to be examined in this section include measures of intelligence, vocabulary, ability to interpret cause-effect relationships, problem solving, divergent thinking, and conservation.

'Intelligence'. The use of representational processes is an important factor in successful performance on many intelligence tests. Therefore, to the extent that training in pretend play facilitates development of representational abilities, it should lead to facilitated performance on such tests. Several experiments have examined this issue.

The most extensive training occurred in the study by *Saltz* et al. [1977]. Training lasted for 6 months, with three sessions per week. Three types of pretend play were examined: sociodramatic, thematic fantasy, and story discussion. In addition, a 'cut and paste' control group was exposed to the experimenters in an emotionally warm environment for an equivalent number of sessions. The children were primarily from lower SES backgrounds; all attended an excellent preschool which stressed verbal and intellectual stimulation. Thus, the various, specific types of training all occurred within the context of a generally stimulating environment. Further, the study was repeated three times, over 3 successive years, to determine the replicability of the results.

In the first year of this experiment, children were posttested on the Peabody Picture Vocabulary Test; in the next 2 years, French's Pictorial Test of Intelligence was used. In each of the 3 years of the study, both sociodramatic and thematic fantasy play training led to significantly better performance on these tests of intellectual functioning than did story discussion or the control condition. The sociodramatic and thematic fantasy conditions did not differ significantly from each other. Results of an earlier pilot study by *Saltz and Johnson* [1974] also indicated a tendency for prolonged thematic fantasy play training to facilitate intellectual performance.

What 'alternative hypotheses' could be offered to account for the effects obtained by *Saltz* et al. [1977] and *Saltz and Johnson* [1974]? Earlier we suggested that familiarity and rapport between experimenter and children being tested is an important factor that must be kept the same for experimental and control conditions. Children in the various conditions of this experiment were exposed to the experimenters approximately equally; this makes unlikely the alternative hypothesis that differences in rapport can account for the obtained differences in intelligence test scores. Another alternative hypothesis is one suggested by *Smith and Syddall* [1978]. These writers suggest that training for pretend play typically involves a relatively large amount of verbal stimulation. If the control conditions do not involve corresponding amounts of verbal stimulation, an alternative hypothesis might be that any superiority in cognitive functioning for the pretend play conditions might be attributable to verbal stimulation, rather than other aspects of pretend play. Control for verbal stimulation was the rationale for including the story discussion condition in the *Saltz* et al. [1977] experiment. In this condition, the children encounter the same type of verbal stimulation as in the thematic fantasy play condition, but without the play activity. The children in the story discussion condition performed significantly below the children in the two play conditions; further, they performed no better than the children in the 'cut and paste' control condition, which involved relatively little verbal stimulation from the experimenters. Finally, the total amount of verbal exchange between experimenters and children in any of the experimental conditions was a small fraction of the verbal exchange between the children and the staff of the preschool. Thus, verbal stimulation does not appear to be a viable alternative hypothesis for the effects of pretend play on intelligence test performance in the *Saltz* et al. [1977] study.

Smith and Syddall [1978] attempted to test the notion that the effects of sociodramatic play training on intelligence test performance are attributable to the verbal stimulation involved in the training for sociodramatic play. One group of 7 preschoolers was trained in sociodramatic play, another group of 7 was trained in various skills activities (e.g., clay modelling). Training lasted 5 weeks, three sessions per week. Both groups showed a significant increase in performance on two tests which are usually interpreted as indices of intelligence, the Caldwell Preschool Inventory and the Draw a Man test. The increase in scores was not significantly different for the sociodramatic play as opposed to the skills training groups. Further, amount of verbal interaction between experimenter and children was monitored during training, and was found to be similar for the two groups. *Smith and Syddall* [1978] interpreted their data as indicating that the observed increases in intelligence test performance for the two groups was due to verbal stimulation; the absence of a difference in intelligence test performance between the two groups was attributed to the fact that verbal stimulation was equated for the groups. Sociodramatic play was interpreted as providing no unique variance to these test scores beyond the occurrence of verbal stimulation in the course of this play.

There are several problems in interpreting the *Smith and Syddall* [1978] study. First, the pre- and postdifferences in intelligence test scores cannot easily be attributed to verbal stimulation since the study did not involve an appropriate control for the alternative hypothesis that rapport, rather than verbal stimulation, produced the observed increases (viz., a control group was needed which was exposed to the experimenters in a friendly manner, but with relatively little verbal stimulation). Indeed, *Smith and Syddall* [1978] found widespread improvement between pre- and posttest measures across a number of different tasks, like intelligence and vocabulary, that usually do not show such large increases over such short intervals. As for the absence of a difference in intelligence test scores between groups, the short length of training and the small number of subjects casts some doubt on the generality of the findings.

In short, three studies have examined the effects of training for pretend play on subsequent performance on standardized tests of intelligence. Two report significant effects as a consequence of pretend play, one does not. The two that found significant effects involved relatively protracted training over 4- to 6-months, and with 30–150 children as subjects. The one that found no effect involved 5 weeks of training with only 7 children in each condition.

Story Integration Test. Young children have a tendency to react to sequences of events as though each event was relatively independent, without perceiving the relationship between them. *Saltz* et al. [1977] developed a Story Integration Test as a measure of the ability of children to relate events in sequences of pictures. Children in the story-discussion condition and in the control condition showed virtually no tendency to integrate sequences. Both thematic fantasy training and sociodramatic training facilitated ability to integrate sequences, but the effects of thematic fantasy training were significantly greater than for sociodramatic play training, and the magnitude of this difference was quite large.

A comparison of the data for story interpretation with the previously summarized data for intelligence indicates a very important difference (a difference that will be encountered again when we consider the data for perspective taking and for impulse control). While training children for thematic fantasy play and for sociodramatic play had equivalent effects on the tests of intelligence, these two types of play did not have equivalent effects on the ability to integrate a sequence of events into a story. This suggests that no single, underlying factor is basic to the different effects on cognitive functioning produced by various pretend-play activities. Some complex of variables must be at work, and these variables do not act in concert for all dependent cognitive functions.

Language Effects. Language variables include word knowledge, syntactic comprehension, and complexity of language structure. Both vocabulary size and the ability to use and comprehend complex sentences relate strongly to general cognitive effectiveness. We have already seen that *Saltz* et al. [1977] found that training in both thematic fantasy play and sociodramatic play led to facilitated vocabulary development as measured by the Peabody Picture Vocabulary Test. On the other hand, *Smith and Syddall* [1978] found no difference between their sociodramatic group and their control group on a composite score based on vocabulary and comprehension subtests of the Reynell Language Development Scale. As was noted earlier, the failure of *Smith and Syddall* [1978] to find significant differences between groups on a factor like vocabulary, which develops slowly, may not be surprising in view of the relatively short training period and the small number of subjects.

Turning to sentence usage, *Freyberg* [1973] reports that training on sociodramatic play led to the use of longer, more complex sentences. *Lovinger* [1974] reports that sociodramatic play training led to superior scores on the Verbal Expression subtest of the Illinois Test of Psycholinguistic Ability (ITPA), as well as to a significant increase in number of words and sentences used in free play. *Lovinger's* [1974] test results on the ITPA are difficult to interpret, since her control group received no intervention training, and therefore probably did not have as much rapport with the tester as the sociodramatic play group. On the other hand, the increased sentence length and number of words used in free play in both of these studies are not likely to be attributable to such rapport differences. Neither study involved control groups that would permit us to evaluate the hypothesis that the obtained differences might have been found with any other training procedure which also encouraged a great deal of verbal interaction.

Problem-Solving and Originality. To the extent that pretend play fosters representational ability, it should facilitate problem-solving and originality. Unfortunately, most of the tasks that measure such activities are too difficult for the young children involved in most of the studies under review in the present chapter. *Rosen* [1974] reports that training in sociodramatic play facilitates group problem-solving. *Feitelson and Ross* [1973] report that such training fosters originality of thinking. And *Dansky* [1980] reports that encouraging such play leads to improved performance on a version of the 'Uses' test for original thinking.

Problem-solving in *Rosen's* [1974] study consisted of a group project in which children were to cooperate in constructing some object. In the best of circumstances, it would not be clear if superior performance on this task by the trained children represented greater socialization, or greater problem-solving ability for individual children. This problem is aggravated in the *Rosen* [1974] study by the fact that the sociodramatically trained children received 40 training sessions, while the control received only 10 sessions, one per week. Thus, rapport has not been convincingly controlled.

Feitelson and Ross [1973] administered only 10 training sessions to the children in their study and the sample size was small (6 children per condition). Despite this, the experiment was well controlled in other respects. In addition to an 'imaginative play' condition, three contrast conditions were employed: (a) 10 sessions of individual instruction on how to play the tonette, a condition which must have involved both a great deal of personal attention plus verbal interaction; (b) sessions in which children were permitted to play with toys in the presence of the experimenter but no tutoring in play occurred; (c) no intervention, only pre- and posttesting. The play group significantly exceeded the other three in 'originality' on Torrance's 'Thinking Creatively with Pictures' test. This score represents number of unusual titles the children will invent for the pictures. The groups did not differ on two other scores for this test: fluency and flexibility. If rapport or verbal stimulation was the critical variable, we would have expected that the originality scores of the children given the individual training on the tonette should have been superior to the scores of the children in the control condition involving no intervention. No tendency in this direction was observed. However, one must wonder what type of ability for original thinking can be developed in a generalized fashion (from play to picture naming) over eight training sessions. *Wallach and Kogan* [1965] have suggested that much of originality may consist of the 'set' or willingness to respond in ways that are different. It seems more reasonable to believe that play could have affected 'set' in such a small number of sessions than that it modified the ability to think of original responses.

The problem of amount of training necessary to affect originality becomes even more troubling in *Dansky's* [1980] study. Here significant effects of play were found after a single 10-min session. He identified children who were likely to engage spontaneously in pretend play. The children were then shown a set of objects (e.g., paperclips, pipe cleaners, etc.) in one of the following conditions: free-play, where a pair of children could play any way they wished with the object; modeling, in which the experimenter modeled innovative activities with the objects; or a problem-solving task involving the objects in which the experimenter provided verbal cues and the children tried to find the answer. Immediately after these treatments, children were shown four new objects (e.g., screwdriver) and asked to indicate all the uses they could for each object. The children in the free-play condition were greatly (and significantly) superior to those in the other conditions. The results cannot easily be attributed to inhibition produced by the modeling or the problem-solving conditions, as is shown by the fact that a no-intervention control performed at about the same level on the Uses test as the other control conditions.

Again, it is difficult to believe that 10 min of experience in playing with one set of objects would increase the general creative ability of children. This is particularly an issue in the *Dansky* [1980] study since the children involved were selected because of their prior propensity for engaging in spontaneous pretend play outside of the intervention situation.

Perhaps the most conservative interpretation of data such as those of *Feitelson and Ross* [1973] and of *Dansky* [1980], is that pretend play tends to prime or 'set' the children to think in more original fashions. Many issues remain unanswered. How persistent are the obtained effects? Are there sizeable individual differences in the effects, as suggested by *Dansky* [1980]? Does practice produce an alteration in the ability to respond creatively, or does it trigger tendencies previously in existence for children who are already relatively creative?

Conservation of Physical and Social Concepts. Piaget's [1932] observation that preschool children are very seldom capable of solving problems involving quantitative invariance has been supported by a great deal of research in almost every corner of the world. *Piaget* [1932] has suggested that one reason for this difficulty is that young children do not understand the principle of reversibility (e.g., if liquid is poured back from a narrow, tall glass to its original wide glass, the water level will be the same as it had been before the water was poured into the narrow, tall glass). *Golomb and Cornelius* [1977] reasoned that reversibility might be taught in the context of pretend play, and might then generalize to conservation problems. In a sequence of three training sessions of about 15 min each, these experimenters trained children in pretend play that emphasized reversibility; e.g., they stressed to the children that a person could take a role, then be himself again when the play ended. The control group spent a corresponding amount of time working puzzles, drawing, and so forth. On a posttest, the pretend play condition significantly exceeded the control in scores on conservation of physical quantity.

Guthrie and Hudson [1979] attempted to replicate the *Golomb and Cornelius* [1977] study as closely as possible, but failed to find the same effect of training on conservation. *Fink* [1976] also failed to find that training on sociodramatic play had an effect on conservation of physical quantity, using eight training sessions of 25 min each. *Fink* [1976] did not, however, appear to stress the reversibility characteristics of pretend play to his young trainees.

The writer would have been surprised had the *Golomb and Cornelius* [1977] findings proven replicable. Conservation seems to develop very slowly during childhood, with relatively little transfer from one type of conservation to another, so that many children can conserve liquid quantity and yet not use the same reversibility argument to understand conservation of weight or volume. It would have been surprising if three training sessions on role reversibility could have transferred to conservation of liquid quantity.

Fink [1976] reports that pretend-play training facilitated performance in the type of task used by *Sigel* et al. [1967], e.g., 'A father goes to work where he is a doctor; is he still a father?' *Sigel* et al. [1967] report that most preschool children feel that a father is no longer a father if he changes roles and becomes a doctor. *Fink's* [1976] data suggest that training in pretend play may facilitate the ability to conserve such social roles in the face of role transformations. Note that conservation of social roles is more similar to pretend-play activities than is conservation of physical quantity.

Role-Taking and Perspective-Taking

Young children tend to be egocentric (i.e., they often do not understand the points of view of other people when these points of view differ from their own). This is true for physical perspectives (e.g., young children often appear surprised to find that their parents, in a different room, do not see what they see); it is also true for social perspectives (e.g., asked what gift mother might like for her birthday, young children may answer tricycle or doll). *Shantz* [1975], in her comprehensive review of the literature on perspective-taking, pointed out that many different tasks have been used as measures of perspective-taking, yet we know relatively little about the relationships between these tasks. Tasks used to measure perspective-taking by one psychologist may be challenged as irrelevant to the concept by another psychologist. Under these circumstances, as *Rubin* [1980] has pointed out, it has become difficult to evaluate the effects of pretend play on perspective-taking. Despite this, a number of psychologists have been interested in the relationship between pretend play and perspective-taking because of the theoretical implications of this relationship [*Chandler*, 1973; *Mead*, 1932; *Smilansky*, 1968].

The relationship between thematic fantasy play and perspective-taking was considered in two studies, those of *Saltz and Johnson* [1974] and *Saltz* et al. [1977]. Both studies used *Borke's* [1973] task as a measure of perspective-taking and in both thematic fantasy play training facilitated performance on the *Borke* [1973] task compared to the performance of the control group. *Saltz* et al. [1977] compared the performance of children trained in thematic fantasy play with that of children trained in sociodramatic play. The authors found that thematic fantasy play led to significantly greater gains in perspective-taking than did sociodramatic training. These were no significant differences between the sociodramatic training and the control groups on the *Borke* [1973] measure.

While *Saltz* et al. [1977] failed to find an effect of sociodramatic play on perspective-taking over a 6-month training period, *Burns and Brainerd* [1979] found an effect over 10 training sessions. These authors measured perspective-taking with a battery of different tasks, and so the children's scores were probably more stable than in most of the other studies in this area. One control condition involved encouraging small groups of children to cooperate over 10 sessions in constructing various specific objects (e.g., house, wagon, or train) using materials provided; children first agreed on the object to construct, then cooperated in the construction. The other control condition merely received pre- and posttests, but no intervention training. On the battery of perspective taking tasks, both the sociodramatic and construction control conditions far exceeded the no-intervention condition. The sociodramatic condition was significantly superior to the construction condition, but the magnitude of this difference was only moderate.

The construction control condition in the *Burns and Brainerd* [1979] study is an interesting and important one. Compared to the sociodramatic condition, it certainly controlled for rapport, and also apparently controlled for the amount of verbal interaction between experimenter and children. Thus, at least part of the superiority of the construction condition over the no-intervention control is probably due to the greater rapport developed over the 10 training sessions. In addition, the cooperative construction play involved interaction between the children; any such cooperative activity is likely to force a certain amount of appreciation of the point of view of others.

In short, cooperative play of any sort, sociodramatic, or fantasy, or construction, is likely to foster some perspective-taking abilities. The *Burns and Brainerd* [1979] study was conducted in a relatively unstimulating daycare setting that was largely custodial in orientation. Against this background, perhaps, almost any amount of encouragement of cooperative activity might have a sizeable impact.

Smith and Syddall [1978] also report a significant facilitation in perspective-taking as a result of training in sociodramatic play. Two perspective-taking tasks taken from *Rosen* [1974] were used. Several other studies have reported significant improvement in perspective-taking as a consequence of training in sociodramatic play [*Fink*, 1976; *Rosen*, 1974]. However, because of methodological problems, the results are difficult to interpret [*Rubin*, 1980].

In conclusion, there is some evidence from *Saltz* et al. [1977] that thematic fantasy play may be more effective than sociodramatic play in fostering perspective-taking skills. In this study, extensive amounts of training on sociodramatic play failed to significantly affect performance on the test used to measure perspective-taking. Why did *Burns and Brainerd* [1979] and *Smith and Syddall* [1978] find that moderate amounts of training on sociodramatic play facilitated perspective taking, while *Saltz* et al. [1977] found no effect after much greater amounts of training? In the case of the *Burns and Brainerd* [1979] study, one reason might be that the measurement of perspective-taking was much more comprehensive and the scores more reliable than in the *Saltz* et al. [1977] study. Another possible reason may be the amount of relevant stimulation in the children's environment outside of the experimental sessions. Given the general lack of stimulation in the daycare setting in which *Burns and Brainerd* [1979] did their research, for example, it is possible that even small amounts of relevant experience might provide a great contrast with the minimal experience of the control children. The background stimulation for the children in *Smith and Syddall's* [1978] study is not known.

Impulse Control

Young children are known to be very stimulus bound; they show little ability to control their responses to the stimuli of the external environment. This results in various types of behavior that are characterized as a lack of impulse control, such as difficulty in delaying gratification. As children develop more complex representational systems, it becomes possible for representational responses to intervene between external stimuli and the immediate firing of motoric responses. This intervention can be assumed to be the basis for impulse control. To the extent that pretend play fosters representational processes, such play should augment impulse control. *Singer* [1961] has presented evidence that children who engage in pretend play are more likely to exhibit waiting behavior.

Unfortunately, most of the evidence on the relationship between pretend play and impulse control comes from one set of experiments, the research of *Saltz* et al. [1974, 1977]. Both the *Saltz and Johnson* [1974] and the *Saltz* et al. [1977] studies examined the effects of thematic fantasy play training on Kagan's MFF test. Both found that fantasy training significantly increased waiting time before making a response. Sociodramatic play training, on the other hand, seemed to have no effect on MFF performance in the *Saltz* et al. [1977] study.

In addition, *Saltz* et al. [1977] examined several situations that permitted children to display their ability to control impulsive behavior. In one situation, children were asked to guard an attractive toy for the experimenter; in another, children were asked to pretend that they were going on a trip to the moon; they were asked not to leave their rocket ship (i.e., their chair) until the ship reached the moon. For both tasks, some children were told to think of something pleasant to take their minds off waiting. Under 'thinking' conditions, training in thematic fantasy play resulted in by far the greatest impulse control; both sociodramatic play, and story-discussion also significantly affected impulse control.

Conclusions

What can we conclude about the effects of pretend play on cognitive functioning? We have seen that training in pretend play leads to improvement in a number of different types of cognitive activities. Could these results be due to the operation of some uncontrolled variable like amount of verbal stimulation, rather than play, per se? In answer to this issue, it must first be noted that the pattern of results appears sufficiently complex that it is unlikely that any single variable is producing all of the effects. For example, thematic fantasy and sociodramatic play training are equally effective in improving vocabulary scores, leading to the conclusion that the critical variable relating play to vocabulary must be approximately equal in these two forms of play. Yet thematic fantasy play appears to be much more effective than sociodramatic play for fostering perspective-taking. Apparently, the aspects of play critical to vocabulary development are not identical to those relevant to the acquisition of perspective-taking.

Smith and Syddall [1978] have suggested that verbal stimulation may be the critical factor in the relationship between play activities and facilitated cognitive functions. The writers fail to find convincing evidence for this suggestion. For example, with regard to perspective-taking, *Smith and Syddall* [1978] themselves found a significant effect even when sociodramatic play and control conditions were monitored to assure equality on this variable. For vocabulary development, the pattern of results in the *Saltz* et al. [1977] study is simply not consistent with the contention that high verbal stimulation alone, led to the obtained differences, even in the absence of pretend play.

Finally, it must be emphasized that there are a great many unanswered questions in the research on pretend play. Often we have seen changes in performance after so few training sessions that it is difficult to believe that basic abilities were altered by the training. How much training is necessary to produce some of the effects of concern? To what extent are reported results the product of priming, rather than changes in skill structure? Almost no follow-up has been reported to determine the stability of any of the observed effects. The season is past for pilot research on the effects of pretend play. Effects have been found. It is now time to examine the bases of these effects.

References

Borke, H.: Interpersonal perception of young children: egocentrism or empathy? Devl Psychol. *5:* 263–269 (1973).

Burns, S.M.; Brainerd, C.J.: Effects of constructive and dramatic play on perspective taking in very young children. Devl Psychol. *15:* 512–521 (1979).

Chandler, M.J.: Egocentrism and antisocial behavior: the assessment and training of social perspective taking skills. Devl Psychol. *8:* 326–332 (1973).

Dansky, J.L.: Make-believe: a mediator in the relationship between play and associative frequency. Child Dev. *51:* 576–579 (1980).

Feitelson, D.; Ross, G.S.: The neglected factor-play. Hum. Dev. *16:* 202–223 (1973).

Fink, R.S.: Role of imaginative play in cognitive development. Psychol. Rep. *39:* 895–906 (1976).

Freyberg, J.: Increasing the imaginative play of urban disadvantaged children through systematic training; in Singer, The child's world of make-believe (Academic Press, New York 1973).

Golomb, C.; Cornelius, C.B.: Symbolic play and its cognitive significance. Devl Psychol. *13:* 246–252 (1977).

Guthrie, K.; Hudson, L.M.: Training conservation through symbolic play: a second look. Child Dev. *50:* 1269–1271 (1979).

Lovinger, S.L.: Sociodramatic play and language development in preschool disadvantaged children. Psychol. Schools *11:* 313–320 (1974).

Mead, G.H.: Mind, self, and society (University of Chicago Press, Chicago 1932).

Piaget, J.: The moral judgement of the child (Free Press, New York 1932).

Rosen, C.E.: The effects of sociodramatic play on problem solving behavior among culturally disadvantaged preschool children. Child Dev. *45:* 920–927 (1974).

Rubin, K.H.: Fantasy play: its role in the development of social skills and social cognition. New Dir. Child Dev. *9:* 69–84 (1980).

Saltz, E.; Dixon, D.; Johnson, J.: Training disadvantaged preschoolers on various fantasy activities: effects on cognitive functioning and impulse control. Child Dev. *48:* 367–380 (1977).

Saltz, E.; Johnson, J.: Training for thematic-fantasy play in culturally disadvantaged children: preliminary results. J. educ. Psychol. *66:* 623–630 (1974).

Shantz, C.U.: The development of social cognition; in Hetherington, Review of child development research, vol. 5 (University of Chicago Press, Chicago 1975).

Sigel, I.E.; Saltz, E.; Roskind, W.: Variables determining concept formation in children. J. exp. Psychol. *74:* 471–475 (1967).

Singer, J.L.: Imagination and waiting ability in young children. J. Personality *29:* 396–413 (1961).

Smilansky, S.: The effects of sociodramatic play on disadvantaged preschool children (Wiley, New York 1968).

Smith, P.K.; Syddall, S.: Play and nonplay tutoring in preschool children: is it play or tutoring which matters? Br. J. educ. Psychol. *48:* 315–325 (1978).

Vygotsky, L.S.: Play and its role in the mental development of the child. Soviet Psychol. *12:* 62–76 (1967).

Wallach, M.A.; Kogan, N.: Modes of thinking in young children (Holt, Rinehart & Winston, New York 1965).

Contr. hum. Dev., vol. 6, pp. 114–129 (Karger, Basel 1982)

Effects of Group and Individualized Dramatic Play Training on Cognitive Development

Charles J. Brainerd[1]

University of Western Ontario, London, Ont., Canada

When it comes to the problems and prospects of play research, the tone of this paper is, I fear, rather more pessimistic than most of the other contributions to this volume. To be precise, it is a paper in which some pessimistic observations are made about learning experiments that seek to improve children's grasp of some familiar concepts by having them participate in play sessions of a particular sort. For the most part, the concepts are ones that we commonly associate with *Piaget's* [1951] concrete-operational stage (e.g., classification, conservation, perspective taking, seriation). The type of play has been variously called dramatic play, fantasy play, pretense play, symbolic play, thematic play, and, I should think, other things as well. Since 'dramatic play' seems to be the most encompassing term, it is the one I shall use here.

The common element in all forms of dramatic play is that children enact the perceived roles of people other than themselves. In learning experiments of the sort that I shall be considering, role enactment usually occurs in a semistructured situation provided by the experimenter or arrived at by mutual agreement between the experimenter and the children. As a rule, the semistructured situation involves small groups of 2 or 3 children. The characters and themes may be from real life – e.g., playing mother or father on a visit to the doctor's office or on a visit to a restaurant – or they may be

[1] Preparation of this paper and the research reported herein were supported by grant No. A0668 from the Natural Sciences and Engineering Research Council. The paper was written while I was on leave at the Institute of Child Development, University of Minnesota.

imaginary – e.g., playing one of the mythical characters in
or in Little Red Riding Hood.

I wish to consider three topics in this paper. First, I
reasons for using training designs to study play in gen
play in particular. These remarks will be brief because a
points are covered elsewhere in this volume. Second, some salient
from a series of experiments published by various investigators during the 1970s and late 1960s will be reviewed. Third, I shall summarize the results of two experiments conducted in my laboratories that were concerned with how dramatic play experience affects young children's performance on various perspective-taking tasks and on conservation problems.

Motivation

The reasons for using learning experiments to study play are both theoretical and empirical. On the theoretical side, we have the claim by *James Mark Baldwin*, *Jean Piaget*, and any number of lesser-known theorists that play is the principal experiential medium in which cognitive development takes place in young children. Here, 'young children' will have its usual meaning of kindergarten down to roughly age 2. I should immediately add that this theoretical claim devolves from an assumption whose validity, at least in retrospect, seems questionable. The assumption is that young children do not yet possess the sheer intellectual hardware that is necessary to benefit from the structured, tutorial learning experiences whereby concepts are commonly transmitted to older children, especially in the classroom [*Brainerd*, 1977, 1978a–c].

Despite a supposed inability to profit from such experiences, during the early childhood years there is clear evidence of age-related improvements in a host of logical, mathematical, physical, and social concepts. Unless we resort to a lazy maturational explanation, we need an experiential mechanism whereby these improvements are effected – hence, the suggestion of play as a possibility.

Although it could certainly be true that play is an important source of cognitive development, the assumption that motivates the hypothesis is evidently wrong. During the past 10–15 years, the structured, tutorial methods that are used to teach concepts to older children have been extensively studied in young children. On the whole, the results have been quite positive. In learning experiments with preschoolers, unmistakable improvements in oncept-test performance have been produced by tutorial procedures such as observation of a skilled model [*Rosenthal and Zimmerman*, 1972], verbal rule instruction [*Denney* et al., 1978], perceptual set training [*Boersma and Wilton*, 1974], and corrective feedback [*Brainerd*, 1974].

Concerning dramatic play per se, the theoretical reason for focusing on this specific form of play grows out of *Piaget's* theory [*Hooper and DeFrain*, 1980]. As everyone knows, *Piaget* thought that young children's lack of conceptual sophistication in many spheres stems from a proclivity to be egocentric. That is, it can be traced to young children's presumed failure to understand that there are points of view – whether physical, intellectual, or social – other than their own. Dramatic play, by definition, consists of enacting the perspectives of other people and behaving accordingly. It is but a small step from this facet of dramatic play to the generalization that extensive participation in such play should reduce children's overall levels of egocentrism. This generalization has prompted some investigators to entertain the idea that dramatic play – as opposed to, say, constructive play, functional play, and other activities that do not incorporate a strong role-taking component – should be closely connected to cognitive development in early childhood.

Once again, I hasten to add that there are grounds for doubting the assumption that underlies this last hypothesis. There is no clear evidence that young children's conceptual difficulties are rooted primarily in egocentrism. Perhaps the most compelling finding is that preschool children are simply not all that egocentric. In the area of language development, for example, it has long been known that egocentric utterances do not predominate in the spontaneous speech of even 2- and 3-year-olds. With respect to other tasks that have served as classic measures of egocentrism – namely, perspective-taking problems – it is true that preschoolers often make errors on such tasks. But it does not now appear that their errors are chiefly the egocentric ones of failing to differentiate the self from other people and objects. *Ford* [1979] has reviewed most of the previous work on this point, and extensive new data are available in a dissertation by *Scheffman* [1981]. At present, then, theories which explain young children's conceptual limitations by relying on other factors, such as space constraints on working memory [*Brainerd*, 1981], seem to be more promising than theories which rely on egocentrism.

There is a final, methodological reason for conducting learning experiments to assess the play/cognitive development relationship. Broadly speaking, the reason is enhanced theoretical interpretability. At first glance, I suppose it would seem that the long-standing antipathy of cognitive-developmental theory to the learning laboratory would preclude the use of learning experiments to study the relationship between cognitive development and *anything*. It does not appear so in this case. It happens that the results of learning experiments are far easier to interpret than those of traditional normative-correlational studies. It might be thought that the obvious research strategy would be to conduct normative-correlational studies using play measures and measures of conceptual knowledge as covariants. Indeed, a number of such studies have been reported, and the pace seems to be accelerating [for a review, see *Rubin*, 1980]. However, establishing that there is or is not covariation between such measures is not very informative. The problem, as *Hintzman* [1980] has recently reminded us in another context, is what statisticians call *Simpson's* [1951] paradox. *Simpson* [1951] showed that, depending on systematic uncontrolled factors (i.e., uncontrolled factors that are related to the dependent variables in some way), the observed relationship between two variables can be positive or negative or zero, regardless of their true relationship in the population. Of course, we have all known since we were undergraduates that two variables, X and Y, which are stochastically independent can be observed to be positively related to some other, uncontrolled variable. This is one aspect of *Simpson's* [1951] paradox. Depending on relationships with uncontrolled variables, two variables can be observed to be negatively related when the true relationship is zero or positive, and they can be observed to be unrelated when the true relationship is positive or negative. Learning experiments are less subject to these psychometric perplexities.

Literature Synopsis

I now turn to the previous literature on how dramatic play experiences affect young children's knowledge of selected concepts. I do not propose to go over the literature study by study. *Rubin* [1980] and *Rubin* et al. [1982] have already done that in recent chapters. Instead, I will summarize what the typical experiment is like and then mention some results that, speaking personally, appear disappointing. These particular findings motivated the experiments to be reported in the next section.

The characteristics of the prototype experiment are as follows. The subjects are kindergarteners or preschoolers, usually the latter. They receive pretests and posttests for concepts from *Piaget's* concrete-operational stage with a dramatic play treatment in between. In nearly all studies, either perspective-taking concepts or conservation concepts have been measured. The reason for selecting perspective taking is its presumptive connection to the role-enactment behavior that goes on in dramatic play. The reason for selecting conservation is simply its presumed centrality in Piagetian theory. The dramatic play treatment consists of several sessions, normally involving small groups of children and of 15–30 min duration. The average number of sessions seems to be in the 6–10 range, with sessions spread over a 1- or 2-week period. In certain experiments, however, the number of sessions has been much greater. For example, *Saltz* et al. [1977] and *Saltz and Johnson* [1974] reported studies in which there were three sessions per week for 6 months. The main question, of course, is whether children who take part in these sessions show better posttest performance on the concept measures when they are compared to controls who show the same level of pretest performance.

Experiments of this type have produced four general results that are rather discouraging and, as I think, do not bode well for the hypothesis that dramatic play is the key source of cognitive development in early childhood. Before mentioning them, however, I should note that this is primarily a literature of one-shot studies rather than cumulative programs of research. It goes without saying that empirical generalization is hazardous in the absence of cumulative research and that we shall not be sure of our facts until we have some more of it. Fortunately, there are signs that this situation may be changing.

Instability of Effects

The first disappointing datum is that, for specific concepts, dramatic-play training has produced learning effects that have proved to be unstable from experiment to experiment, one might even say notoriously so. For example, *Saltz* et al. [1977] did not find improvements in affective perspective taking after 6 months of dramatic-play training, whereas other investigators have [*Burns and Brainerd*, 1979]. Inconsistent results have also been obtained for conservation concepts. In an initial study by *Golomb and Cornelius* [1977], large improvements in quantity conservation were measured after six play sessions. But in a later study by *Golomb and Friedman* [1979], there was no immediate improvement in quantity conservation after the same number of sessions.

An explanation of such failures to replicate that comes immediately to mind is reliability. Perspective-taking tests have been the conceptual measures in the majority of studies, and as *Ford* [1979] has painstakingly documented in his review, there are grounds for doubting the reliability of many of these tests. Although this explanation may apply to perspective-taking experiments, it is not promising when it comes to other failures to replicate. To begin with, it would not seem to be applicable to conservation experiments. The standard tests for those conservation concepts that have been measured in play-training experiments (number and quantity) are known to be highly reliable. The KR-20 and test-retest reliabilities are in the 0.80–0.90 range. Also, the reliability explanation does not apply to those perspective-taking experiments in which the tests were chosen with due regard for reliability. In one of the experiments reported below, for example, satisfactory reliability estimates were obtained for measures of cognitive, affective, and perceptual perspective taking, but there were negligible learning effects.

Internal Inconsistencies

The second disappointing datum, one that is related to the first, has to do with inconsistencies that occur within particular experiments. In most studies, more than one conceptual measure is administered, and the measures correlate positively with each other on the pretest. In other words, they measure the same conceptual skills to a degree. But when learning effects have been observed at all, they have been observed for some of these correlated measures but not others. Worse, there is no apparent reason why play training would be more likely to work for some measures than for others. Internal inconsistencies of this sort have been obtained in earlier studies by *Rosen* [1974], *Saltz* et al. [1977] and *Saltz and Johnson* [1974]. They are also evident in the first experiment reported in the next section. In this experiment, among other measures, two types of cognitive perspective-taking tests and two types of affective perspective-taking tests were administered. A learning effect was observed for one test in each category, but not for the other.

Age Interaction

The third disappointing datum is that the effectiveness of dramatic play as a learning treatment seems to interact with age. The specific age × treatment interaction is what is usually called a diverging fan in the measurement theory literature – i.e., treatment effectiveness increases with age. Actually, age has not been systematically varied in most experiments. However, a comparison of different studies involving the administration of the same concept tests strongly suggests that dramatic play produces more improvement when the subjects are kindergarteners than when they are preschoolers. In the case of conservation concepts, for example, the learning effects reported by *Fink* [1976] with kindergarteners are larger than those that have been reported for preschoolers by *Golomb and Cornelius* [1977]; *Golomb and Friedman* [1979], *Saltz* et al. [1977] and *Saltz and Johnson* [1974], Similarly, in the two experiments reported in the next section, the effects of dramatic play on perspective-taking concepts were larger for preschoolers who were nearing their 5th birthday than for 4-year-olds.

At this point, the reader may be inclined to say, 'So what if learning is more pronounced for kindergarteners? Don't older children learn just about anything more readily than younger children?' Although the answer to the second question is usually yes, this particular age interaction has serious implications for the hypothesis that dramatic play is a causal agent in cognitive development. There are two reasons. First, recall that the theoretical hypothesis we are interested in assumes that play in general and dramatic play in particular are learning media which are peculiarly well-adapted to the capacities of preschoolers. In effect, there is a 'critical period' for profiting from play experience that is localized within early childhood. Hence, it would appear reasonable to expect (a) that dramatic play will produce larger learning effects with younger as opposed to older children and (b) that it will work better than the structured, tutorial procedures favored with older children. Our experiments do not seem to be delivering finding a, and I shall presently argue that we do not get finding b either.

The second reason that this apparent age trend has negative implications is that it raises the possibility that the learning effects observed in those studies where dramatic play has had the greatest impact (i.e., with children above preschool age) are performance effects rather than competence effects. Whenever a subject makes an error on a concept test, there are always two possible explanations – i.e., he or she does not have the concept (a competence explanation) or a false negative error has been committed (a performance explanation). As subjects become older, the probability that the competence explanation is correct decreases and the probability that the performance explanation is correct increases. Consequently, whenever a learning procedure is observed to have significant effects on older children but not on younger children, it can be argued that the procedure does not induce conceptual knowledge per se, but rather, it helps subjects overcome various sources of false negative error (performance deficits).

Size of Effects

The last disappointing datum is the most serious of the four, and it probably explains the first two as well. To be quite plain, the learning effects obtained in play-training experiments are, from a purely quantitative standpoint, tiny. They are tiny both in an absolute sense and in a relative sense. Speaking absolutely, the amount of improvement observed on any given conceptual measure, when improvement is observed at all, has been modest. In *Rosen's* [1974] experiment, for example, children who were given 40 h of dramatic play experience were only 7% better than controls on tests of perceptual perspective-taking.

Speaking relatively, learning effects from dramatic play, when they are observed, are much smaller than those that are typically obtained with other procedures. This is clear for both conservation concepts and perspective-taking concepts. I mentioned earlier that several tutorial methods (e.g., observation of skilled models, corrective feedback) have been studied in learning experiments with young children. In fact, several experiments have been published on each of the more familiar methods, and more important, these methods have been used to train the same concepts as in dramatic-play experiments, namely, various types of perspective-taking and conservation. Suffice it to say that the magnitude of the learning effects that such procedures have produced in preschoolers far exceeds that which has been observed in dramatic-play experiments [*Brainerd*, 1974, 1977, 1978b; *Denney* et al., 1978; *Rosenthal and Zimmerman*, 1972].

If it is true that the improvements in concept-test performance that accrue from dramatic play are very circumscribed, then failures to replicate and internal inconsistencies within individual experiments are inevitable. Whenever a between-group effect is precise (say, on the order of one quarter of the within-group variation), we will frequently fail to observe the effect for statistical reasons, unless extremely large numbers of subjects are run. Thus, failures to replicate may not be 'failures' at all as long as the sampling variation of the study falls within certain boundaries.

Two Experiments

These and other shortcomings of the dramatic-play training literature prompted the two experiments which I now report. In the beginning, the hope was that play-training experiments conducted under more carefully controlled conditions might provide a more optimistic picture than the extant literature. In the event, however, the experiments tended to confirm the four trends discussed in the preceding section.

The Burns and Brainerd Experiment

This experiment was conducted during the summer of 1977, and it has been reported in greater detail elsewhere [*Burns and Brainerd*, 1979]. The subjects were 51 day-care children who would be entering kindergarten in September. The mean age of the group was 4 years and 10 months. 17 subjects (11 boys and 6 girls) were assigned to a dramatic-play training condition, and 17 subjects (11 boys and 6 girls) were assigned to a pretest-posttest control condition. 17 subjects (11 boys and 6 girls) were also assigned to a constructive-play training condition. Although the focus of the study was on dramatic play, constructive play was included as a form of activity that, according to cognitive-developmental theory, should not work as well as dramatic play [*Golomb and Cornelius*, 1977].

The experiment was a standard pretest-training-posttest design. For the dramatic play and constructive play conditions, the experiment consisted of 12 sessions of roughly 20 min duration spread over 3 weeks. The sessions took place on consecutive days, except when weekends intervened. The first and 12th sessions were devoted to administering various tests of perspective-taking concepts. There was one test of perceptual perspective taking, two tests of cognitive perspective taking, and two tests of affective perspective taking. Sessions 2–11 comprised the play treatment. Subjects participated in these sessions in small groups of 2 or 3. In the ten dramatic play sessions, the aim was to have the children engage in the sort of prolonged role enactment that has been described by *Saltz* et al. [1977] and *Saltz and Johnson* [1974]. Some everyday theme was chosen for each session (going to the doctors' office, cooking in the kitchen, etc.). Each day's theme was introduced by the experimenter at the start of the session, and the children decided which roles they wished to take. In the ten constructive play sessions, the aim was to have children attain specific concrete objectives via group effort. At the start of the first session, the experimenter set the goal. In each case, the task was to construct some familiar object (a wagon, a house, etc.) out of play materials that were available in the experimental room. During subsequent sessions, the children decided the object to be constructed.

The control procedure was the same as the procedure for the play conditions, minus the ten play sessions. That is, the control subjects were administered the pretests at the same time as the dramatic and constructive play subjects, and likewise for the posttests.

Table I. Mean posttest scores for the *Burns and Brainerd* [1979] experiment

Concept test	Condition		
	control	constructive play	dramatic play
Perceptual task	0.82	2.00	2.35
Cognitive task No. 1	1.59	2.71	2.82
Cognitive task No. 2	0.00	0.18	0.24
Affective task No. 1	4.29	4.24	4.94
Affective task No. 2	2.35	3.00	3.12

The range of possible scores was 0–2 (cognitive task No. 2), 0–4 (perceptual task, cognitive task No. 1, and affective task No. 2), and 0–6 (affective task No. 1).

The numerical results for the three conditions appear in table I. Since pretest and posttest scores should correlate in all three conditions (assuming that the tests are reliable), the main analysis for learning effects consisted of a series of one-way analyses of covariance, i.e., one analysis for each of the six performance measures plus an analysis for the combined scores. For the combined scores, there was a large between-group effect, $F(2,47) = 30.95$, $p < 0.05$. Decomposition of this effect showed that the mean combined posttest score of the two play conditions was larger than the mean combined posttest score of the control condition, $t(47) = 5.32$, $p < 0.05$. The mean combined posttest score of the dramatic play condition was slightly larger than the mean combined posttest score of the constructive play condition, $t(33) = 2.34$, $p < 0.05$.

The analyses for the individual perspective-taking measures revealed that there were learning effects for the perceptual task, $F(2,47) = 12.02$, $p < 0.05$, for one of the two cognitive tasks, $F(2,47) = 8.53$, $p < 0.05$, and one of the affective tasks, $F(2,47) = 7.32$, $p < 0.05$. For the remaining measures, the posttest performance of the controls was as good as the posttest performance of the children in either play condition.

On the whole, the results of this experiment appear more optimistic for dramatic play training than the data of earlier experiments. However, note that two of the disappointing findings mentioned earlier are also in evidence here. First, there is internal inconsistency in the sense that the two types of play affected some perspective-taking measures but not others. Since the effects were not localized within some particular type of perspective taking (e.g., perceptual versus cognitive and affective), there is no obvious explanation for the inconsistency. Second, the size of the learning effect is still small by the standards of the literature on children's concept learning. When all six tests were combined, the range of possible posttest scores in this experiment was 0–20. As can be seen from table I, the average combined posttest score was 9.06 for controls, 12.06 for constructive play subjects, and 13.41 for dramatic play subjects. Thus, the overall learning effect amounted to 3 points on a 20-point scale for constructive play and $4^1/_3$ points on a 20-point scale for dramatic play.

The Scheffman Experiment

The next experiment, a doctoral project by *Scheffman* [1981], grew out of the results of *Burns and Brainerd* [1979]. Essentially, the aims were the familiar ones of replication and extension. More specifically, *Scheffman* [1981] hoped to produce more substantial learning effects by including a broader range of concept tests, by giving more careful consideration to the reliability of the individual measures, and by modifying the dramatic-play procedure for trained subjects.

The subjects were 75 day-care children whose mean age was 4 years and 0 months. The experiment was conducted during the fall of 1979, and obviously, the children were 1 year younger than those in the preceding experiment. *Scheffman* [1981] expanded the design of the *Burns and Brainerd* [1979] experiment in three ways. First, she included more treatment combinations. The control, group-dramatic play, and group-constructive play conditions were again included. The procedures for the two play conditions (pretests followed by ten play sessions followed by posttests) and for the control condition (pretest followed by posttests) were the same as before. However, an individualized dramatic-play condition and an individualized constructive-play condition were added to the design. The procedures for each of these individualized conditions were the same as for the corresponding group condition, except that each subject played individually with the experimenter rather than in small groups. The idea behind the individualized play method was that it might be possible to produce much larger learning effects than in the *Burns and Brainerd* [1979] experiment if the children were engaged in one-on-one play with an adult. See *Scheffman* [1981] for a discussion of the rationale that underlies this hypothesis.

The second expansion was to include more concept tests, in the hope that some sensible relationship between size of learning effects and type of concept measured would begin to emerge. The five perspective-taking tests administered by *Burns and Brainerd* [1979] were also administered by *Scheff-*

man [1981]. In addition, a third test of cognitive perspective taking, three tests of referential communication, a second test of perceptual perspective taking, and a number-conservation test were administered, for a total of eleven concept tests in all.

The third expansion was to conduct a detailed analysis of both the test-retest and internal reliabilities of the various measures. The analysis of test-retest reliability was based on a separate sample of 37 children from the same day-care centers as the children in five experimental conditions. These subjects were given an initial administration of the eleven concept tests, followed by a readministration 2 weeks later. The analysis of internal reliability was based on the pretest administration of the concept-test battery to the 75 children in the main experimental conditions. Here, the motivation was that a detailed study of reliability might reveal clear relationships between size of learning effects and reliability of dependent variables.

When it comes to the question of how powerful dramatic (and constructive) play is as an enhancer of conceptual knowledge, the results were extremely disappointing. For all intents and purposes, there were no learning effects. The principal analysis for learning effects consisted of a series of 12 one-way analyses of covariance (one for each concept test plus one for total scores on the battery as a whole). Only one of these analyses (for one of the perceptual perspective-taking tasks) produced a null hypothesis rejection. Since there were 12 tests in all, a single null hypothesis rejection is about what one would expect by chance. The picture did not change when various training groups were combined. For example, the pooled posttest performance for the two dramatic-play treatments was not better than the posttest performance of the controls. Similarly, the pooled posttest performance for the two constructive-play treatments was not better than the posttest performance of the controls.

Turning to the reliability analysis, the obvious hypothesis is that the absence of learning effects is due to the low reliability of the measures. However, the reliability data reported in table II afford no support for this hypothesis. Although the test-retest and/or internal reliabilities of some measures are rather low, for the most part the values are satisfactory. Hence, it appears that we must look elsewhere for an explanation of the discrepancy between *Burns and Brainerd's* [1979] learning effects and *Scheffman's* [1981].

There is another point about the correlational data for the concept tests that is of passing interest, namely, predictive validity. In a recent review, *Ford* [1979] has challenged the construct validity of the concept of egocentrism on the ground that tests of the basic forms of egocentrism do not

Table II. Reliabilities of the 11 measures in the *Scheffman* [1981] experiment

Measure	Type of reliability	
	test-retest	internal (alpha)
1 Perceptual task No. 1	0.48	0.68
2 Perceptual task No. 2	0.48	0.53
3 Cognitive task No. 1	0.64	0.39
4 Cognitive task No. 2	0.64	0.79
5 Cognitive task No. 3	0.26	0.61
6 Affective task No. 1	0.74	0.40
7 Affective task No. 2	0.51	0.55
8 Referential task No. 1	0.74	0.86
9 Referential task No. 2	0.72	0.94
10 Referential task No. 3	0.61	0.94
11 Number conservation	0.81	0.58

correlate very well with each other. But as he also notes, most of the available evidence involves two or three concept tests. There does not appear to be any published study in which multiple measures of all four types of egocentrism (perceptual, cognitive, affective, and linguistic) have been administered to the same subjects. In the *Scheffman* [1981] study, however, all four types of egocentrism were studied and there was more than one measure of each type. Hence, the study provides quite comprehensive evidence on the relationship between different domains of egocentrism.

The relevant correlations are shown in table III. Two general patterns emerge. First, with certain exceptions, the tests within a domain tend to correlate with each other – i.e., they seem to define a dimension of some sort. Second, the tests within a domain do not tend to correlate with tests in any other domain. Thus, although the tests in each category are reasonably reliable, they do not seem to be measures of the same construct, as was once supposed.

Three of the treatments in *Scheffman's* [1981] experiment (group dramatic play, group constructive play, and control) were the same as corresponding treatments in *Burns and Brainerd's* [1979] experiment. Apart from the fact that six more concept tests were administered in *Scheffman's* experiment, these three conditions were point-for-point replications of *Burns and Brainerd*. And yet, there was no evidence of learning. Since the only variable on which the experiments differed systematically was age, the fact that *Scheffman's* subjects were roughly 1 year younger than *Burns and Brainerd's* is the only plausible explanation of the discrepancy in learning effects.

Table III. Correlation matrix for the 11 measures in the *Scheffman* [1981] experiment

Measure	Measure 1	2	3	4	5	6	7	8	9	10	11
1		0.53	0.07	0.17	0.08	0.17	0.04	–0.02	0.00	–0.03	–0.15
2			–0.05	0.17	–0.04	0.18	–0.08	–0.01	0.01	0.00	–0.13
3				0.00	–0.13	0.09	0.01	0.07	0.32	0.19	–0.07
4					0.03	0.12	0.08	0.01	–0.06	–0.14	–0.14
5						0.10	0.86	0.15	0.09	0.14	–0.01
6							0.28	0.35	0.33	0.34	0.10
7								0.29	0.27	0.29	0.13
8									0.26	0.19	0.20
9										0.86	–0.03
10											–0.03
11											

n = 75 for this analysis. The numbering of the dependent variables is the same as in table II.

Play in the Preschool

Although theoretical concerns have been emphasized in this paper, there is a practical point about curriculum development that arises from these data. For the past several years, there has been vigorous development of preschool curricula based on Piagetian ideas. Recently, debates have ensued as to which of these new curricula is the most devout rendering of Holy Writ [*Hooper and DeFrain*, 1980]. A standard theme in such curricula is the intensive use of play, especially dramatic play, to promote conceptual growth. But to the extent that the aim of the preschool experience is to transmit concepts or to enhance the probability of their acquisition, the data of play-learning experiments are signalling us that dramatic play is a poor way to do the job. It has simply not produced the sorts of robust learning effects that would be required to justify its widespread use, even in the experiments of *Saltz* et al. [1977] and *Saltz and Johnson* [1974] where there were hundreds of hours of dramatic play.

These results need not be a cause for despair among early childhood educators, however. The experimental analysis of young children's concept learning has identified a number of alternative methodologies that generate good learning in the sense of large improvements in target concepts, good retention across time, and transfer to related concepts [*Brainerd*, 1978a, b].

It must be added that things are clearcut only if the goal of a preschool curriculum is to promote conceptual growth in areas that adults deem to be important. If, on the other hand, the goal is to promote social competence, emotional development, or the general well-being of the child, other techniques will probably be necessary, and dramatic play may be an appropriate choice. But I know of no positive evidence to suggest that this is so. Although some correlational evidence is available on the relationship between various types of play and socioemotional development [*Rubin* et al., in press], the relevant learning experiments have not yet been done.

References

Boersma, F.; Wilton, K.M.: Eye movements and conservation acceleration. J. exp. Child Psych. *17:* 49–60 (1974).

Brainerd, C.J.: Training and transfer of transitivity, conservation, and class inclusion of length. Child Dev. *45:* 324–334 (1974).

Brainerd, C.J.: Cognitive development and concept learning: an interpretative review. Psychol. Bull. *84:* 919–939 (1977).

Brainerd, C.J.: Piaget's theory of intelligence (Prentice-Hall, Englewood Cliffs 1978a).

Brainerd, C.J.: Learning research and Piagetian theory; in Siegel, Brainerd, Alternatives to Piaget: critical essays on the theory, pp. 69–109 (Academic Press, New York 1978b).

Brainerd, C.J.: Cognitive development and instructional theory. Con. educ. Psych. *2* (1978c).

Brainerd, C.J.: Working memory and the developmental analysis of probability judgment. Psychol. Rev. (in press 1981).

Burns, S.M.; Brainerd, C.J.: Effects of constructive and dramatic play on perspective taking in very young children. Devl Psychol. *15:* 512–521 (1979).

Denny, N.W.; Zeytinoglu, S.; Selzer, C.: Conservation training in four-year-old children. J. exp. Child Psych. *24:* 129–146 (1978).

Fink, R.S.: Role of imaginative play in cognitive development. Psychol. Rep. *39:* 895–906 (1976).

Ford, M.: The construct validity of egocentrism. Psychol. Bull. *86:* 1169–1188 (1979).

Golomb, C.; Cornelius, C.: Symbolic play and its cognitive significance. Devl Psychol. *13:* 246–252 (1977).

Golomb, C.; Friedman, L.: Play and cognition: a study of pretense play and conservation of quantity (unpubl. manuscript 1979).

Hintzman, D.L.: Simpson's paradox and the analysis of memory retrieval. Psychol. Rev. *87:* 398–410 (1980).

Hooper, F.H.; DeFrain, J.D.: On delineating distinctly Piagetian contributions to education. Genet. Psychol. Monogr. *101:* 151–181 (1980).

Piaget, J.: Play, dreams, and imitation in childhood (Norton, New York 1951).

Rosen, C.E.: The effects of sociodramatic play on problem-solving behavior among culturally disadvantaged preschool children. Child Dev. *45:* 920–927 (1974).

Rosenthal, T.L.; Zimmerman, B.J.: Modeling by exemplification and instruction in training conservation. Devl Psychol. *6:* 392–401 (1972).

Rubin, K.H.: Fantasy play: its role in the development of social skills and social cognition; in Rubin, Children's play (Jossey-Bass, San Francisco 1980).

Rubin, K.H.; Fein, G.G.; Vandenberg, B.: Play; in Hetherington, Handbook of child psychology: social development (Wiley, New York in press 1982).

Saltz, E.; Dixon, D.; Johnson, J.: Training disadvantaged preschoolers on various fantasy activities: effects on cognitive functioning and impulse control. Child Dev. *48:* 367–380 (1977).

Saltz, E.; Johnson, J.: Training for thematic-fantasy play in culturally disadvantaged children: preliminary results. J. educ. Psychol. *66:* 623–630 (1974).

Scheffman, J.H.: The effects of individual and group play experiences on preschooler's perspective-taking, referential communication, and number conservation abilities; unpubl. doctoral diss. University of Western Ontario (1981).

Simpson, E.H.: The interpretation of interaction in contingency tables. Jl statist. Soc. *13:* 238–241 (1951).

Contr. hum. Dev., vol. 6, pp. 130–143 (Karger, Basel 1982)

Curricular Effects on the Play of Preschoolers

James E. Johnson, Joan Ershler

University of Wisconsin-Madison, Madison, Wisc., USA

Although considerable research has been conducted over the past two decades evaluating the effects of preschool curricula on cognitive development, the impact of different preschool programs on children's play behaviors has been to a great extent less thoroughly investigated. This is unfortunate since play behaviors and cognitive abilities may be reciprocally related, with the effectiveness of more formalized instructional components of a preschool program depending at least in part on what children do during free play periods. For instance, if small group instruction in a preschool is intended to foster specific cognitive skills, behaviors performed by children during free play many or may not involve those skills. If they do, then whatever benefits the small group training has on cognitive development could be amplified or even multiplied over time as a result of the children practicing on their own the skills acquired in the small groups. Documenting curricular effects on free play behaviors, then, would seem necessary both for providing more detailed, comprehensive descriptions of preschool curricula, as well as for providing formative evaluation of programs.

At the same time, one can understand why researchers have paid more attention to cognitive rather than noncognitive outcomes in assessing the effects of preschool programs. Compared to noncognitive outcomes such as play behaviors, cognitive outcomes of preschool programs often are more traceable to specific antecedent factors in the environment. That is, instructional components of the preschool curriculum, from structured large or small group activities to individualized tutorials, represent learning arrangements that are fairly standard with a content often corresponding closely to the content of the cognitive measures used in the outcome evaluation.

In contrast, it would appear more difficult to determine the correspondences between aspects of a given curriculum and preschool play behaviors. Children at play, by definition, do or should have wide latitude in their choice of activities and use of materials. Hence, the gap between what constitutes the 'effective' or actual curriculum as opposed to the 'formal' or intended curriculum can be quite wide for this behavioral domain. Nevertheless, while the degree of latitude in selecting activities may itself be an important curricular dimension, understanding how objects, materials, and teacher behaviors directly or indirectly influence play would seem to be a necessary step in linking the overall curriculum to particular forms of preschool play.

Additional insight into the mechanisms by which curricular effects on play are achieved may be gained by examining how preschool teachers manage time and space in sequencing and organizing daily activities and events [*Darvill*, this volume; *Phyfe-Perkins*, 1980]. Likewise, although more difficult to define and measure, classroom atmosphere and teaching attitudes and values also warrant scrutiny as factors which can affect children's play. These factors may be observed in the subtle forms of verbal and nonverbal classroom interactions between teachers and preschool children. Finally, the effect of the curriculum on play can be expected to vary depending upon the preschool child's age, gender, social class, ethnic background and family constellation. In addition, curricular effects may interact with the child's play predispositions which emanate, in part, from parental socialization practices and attitudes. Given these conceptual and methodological problems, it may not seem too surprising that relatively little empirical work has attempted to measure the impact of the preschool curriculum on the play behavior of young children.

Differences in Preschool Curricula

Conceptualizing a Continuum of Preschool Programs

One way to conceptualize preschool programs is to place them on a continuum representing degree of structure. Degree of structure for present purposes is defined by the extent of teacher-led activities in the classroom and by the relative importance given by the teacher to convergent as opposed to divergent types of thinking. Teacher-led activities refer to those activities in which the teacher plays a prevalent role in directing children's behaviors. Children are expected to accommodate to the teacher's objectives. Convergent learning activities involve the use of materials and teacher performance designed to elicit from children responses directed toward the solving of problems that have one solution or answer (e.g., teacher's use of closed questions). Divergent learning experiences, on the other hand, result from the teacher's use of various activities and problems in a more open-ended way, accepting from children a variety of appropriate responses and answers (e.g., teacher's use of open-ended questions). Highly structured preschool programs are those with a preponderance of teacher-led activities with a strong emphasis on convergent learning, while less structured programs are more child-centered with curricular emphasis on divergent as well as convergent learning. Less structured programs can be viewed as more intellectually risk-free, encouraging creativity in thought and action. This definition of curriculum structure compares with that of *Hess and Croft* [1972]. In their view, more highly structured preschool programs tend to emphasize cognitive skills acquisition, content learning, didactic instruction, and extrinsic motivation, while less structured programs tend to emphasize the social and emotional well-being and development of the child, cognitive processes, learning by discovery, and intrinsic motivation.

In practice, different preschool models fall somewhere along a continuum of structure. For example, a program with a very high level of structure is the *Bereiter and Engelmann* [1966] program with its use of patterned drills, teacher modelling, and controlled or limited use of play-things. Close in degree of structure would be the *Montessori* [1964] program with its carefully programmed activities and didactic play materials. At the other end of the continuum would be traditional or child-centered programs that tend to encourage a variety of play experiences, such as pretend games, physical exercise activities, and manipulative play [Rainbow Series, 1965]. A program with an intermediate amount of structure is the DARCEE curriculum [*Cupp*, 1967] that emphasizes content with the level of structure tending to be uniform throughout the daily schedule. Careful attention to curriculum content and the combination of formal and informal teaching also is characteristic of neo-Piagetian programs [*Ammon*, 1977].

Views on Play Development

Play development during the preschool years has been assumed to occur along both social and cognitive dimensions. *Parten* [1932] suggested the following social play stages: unoccupied, solitary, onlooker, parallel, associative, and cooperative. 3-year-olds were viewed by *Parten* to engage in primarily unoccupied or onlooker activity or solitary play, 4-year-olds in primarily parallel play, and 5-year-olds in primarily associative or cooperative play. However, *Parten's* original formulation is suspect in at least two ways. First, evidence is available that solitary play is not age-related, as stated by her. Rather than being a sign of social immaturity, solitary play is displayed in both younger and older preschoolers, the latter playing alone usually in a constructive or educational way [*Moore* et al., 1974; *Rubin* et al., 1976, 1978]. Secondly, *Parten's* [1932] statement that parallel play is an intermediate play stage has come under attack. Researchers have reported nonsignificant age effects on parallel play [*Bakeman and Brownlee*, 1980; *Johnson and Ershler*, 1981; *Rubin and Krasnor*, 1980; *Smith*, 1977]. *Smith* [1977] found that 2- and 3-year-olds went directly from solitary play to group play without showing a tendency for parallel play. He suggested that parallel play might be an optional play stage. *Bakeman and Brownlee* [1980] detected in their sequential analysis of ongoing play behavior that 3-year-olds typically exhibit parallel play as a bridge to social play. They concluded that parallel play may represent a transient adjustment to a social situation but may not be the hallmark of a developmental stage.

Piaget [1962] outlined the following stages of play in early cognitive development: practice play, symbolic play and games-with-rules, corresponding to the sensorimotor, preoperational, and concrete operational stages of intellectual growth, respectively. *Smilansky* [1968] adapted *Piaget's* [1962] play stages for studying the play of preschoolers. She defined functional play as the routine and stereotypic use of play materials or simple motoric activity, constructive play as sequential and purposeful behavior resulting in a finished product, and dramatic play as thematic role play entailing the transformation of situations or objects. *Smilansky* [1968] found constructive play to be very common in preschool classrooms and viewed this behavior to be a transitional form of play preceding dramatic play. Sociodramatic play (i.e., persistent and communicative pretense in a group), *Smilansky* felt, was the highest play attainment of preschoolers. However, whether a preschooler opts for imaginative play over more reality-based play activities may depend more on personality factors than on the forces of development [*Singer*, 1973].

Although different views have been expressed as to the order, end state, and relationships among the social and cognitive play stages, researchers and practitioners alike have used the play categories of *Parten* [1932] and *Smilansky* [1968] either independently or in combination. The recommendation that social and cognitive play scales be used conjointly is supported by research demonstrating that some social class and age differences in play remain concealed unless play behavior is viewed within the perspective of nested social-cognitive play scales of *Parten* and *Smilansky* [*Rubin* et al., 1976, 1978].

Studies of Preschool Curricula and Play

In their monograph describing the dimensions and effects of four preschool programs, *Miller and Dyer* [1975] stated that the play effects of a program model can be seen most clearly in the criteria for the selection of toys and materials. While here we are concerned primarily with play behavior, it is interesting to note that in two of the programs they studied, the *Montessori* [1964] and *Bereiter and Engelmann* [1966] programs, each set of materials for children's activities was intended to teach one concept. As *Bereiter and Engelmann* [1966, p. 72] stated: 'A good toy does not teach a little bit of everything. If it is good, it is a good vehicle for *one* concept. It should be presented in such a way that the child learns this concept.' This view is antithetical to child-development-oriented programs. Toy selection guidelines for the traditional programs have stated: 'Toys should be abstract; that is, they should look not too literally like any specific object' [Rainbow Series, 1965].

Miller and Dyer [1975] observed 214 children who averaged 4 years of age and who were from economically oppressed families. The children were enrolled in 14 classrooms in ten schools that represented four preschool models. Assessment for the most part consisted of cognitive and noncognitive testing. Teacher ratings of the children's behavior were also available. The authors reported that in the most structured programs (i.e., the Bereiter-Engelmann and Montessori programs), there was less role play but higher amounts of verbal recitation than in DARCEE and traditional programs. Role play was most prevalent, by far, in the traditional programs. On the other hand, manipulative activity with materials was most common in the Montessori programs, followed by the traditional, Bereiter and Engelmann, and DARCEE programs, in that order.

Additional research has been done on the play of children enrolled in Montessori preschool programs that is consistent with the *Miller and Dyer* [1975] findings. *Beller* et al. [1971], using a specially devised Piagetian coding scheme for play, found that Montessori children engaged in significantly less symbolic play and in significantly more practice play behavior than children of the same age who were enrolled in either traditional or open preschools. Children attending the open classrooms exhibited the most symbolic and the least practice play of all. Findings of a more recent study by *Rubin and Bryant* [reported in *Rubin and Seibel*, 1979] are also consistent with these results. *Rubin and Bryant* found that preschoolers attending Montessori programs were often seen performing solitary and constructive-parallel play, but were significantly less often observed in functional- and dramatic-cooperative play. It is interesting that these play behavior descriptions of children enrolled in Montessori preschool programs agree with the test results of *Dreyer and Rigler* [1969], who showed that Montessori children were more task oriented but less creative than preschoolers attending child-development-oriented programs. Still, *Griffing* [1980] observed that higher SES black children in Montessori kindergartens, when given an opportunity, performed very imaginatively in semistructured play situations even though sociodramatic play was not part of their everyday curriculum. Apparently, a little encouragement can go a long way. Curricular effects seem to pertain to play performance, not competence.

Huston-Stein et al. [1977] investigated the relationship of classroom structure to social and play behaviors of 141 economically impoverished preschool children. Children who averaged 4 years and 2 months of age attended one of 13 classrooms. As in the *Miller and Dyer* [1975] study, both classroom dimensions and the children's behaviors were measured. Data were collected over a 5-month period using a time-sampling procedure and a coding system consisting of a list of categories indexing both the children's and the teacher's behaviors. The classroom structure was operationalized by the number of teacher-led activities and by rating scores assessing teacher's warmth and support, harsh discipline, and program structure. Using classroom size and children's ethnicity as control variables, analyses revealed that children in less structured classes were more likely to display imaginative play than those in highly structured programs, even though children in the former programs tended to engage in slightly less positive social interaction than those in the latter programs. Although the findings were correlational, the authors concluded that classroom structure more likely determined children's behavior than vice versa. For example, low levels of fantasy play by children would seem unlikely to stimulate high classroom structure, but high structure may facilitate behaviors in children such as attention to tasks and conformity to adults. The authors concluded that while a structured program may result in cognitive gains for disadvantaged children, it may be doing so at the expense of overlooking the potential value of imaginative play as a vehicle for fostering cognitive abilities, social skills, and positive affect.

Tizard et al. [1976] observed the play of 109 3- and 4-year-old children attending 12 English preschool classes – four classrooms representing each of three types of programs: (1) traditional English nursery schools staffed by trained nursery school teachers; (2) nursery school classrooms like the above but with an added language enrichment component, and (3) nurseries without trained staff or a language enrichment component. The children's use of materials and the social and organizational level of their play was monitored during free play periods. Analyses were conducted to determine the effects of center type, social class, and the child's gender on play behavior. Across social classes, the play of children enrolled in the language enrichment centers was different from that of children in the traditional programs in two ways. First, there was more symbolic play and less 'appropriate' (functional) play in the enrichment classrooms than in the traditional classrooms. Second, in the enrichment programs both working class and middle class preschoolers showed more frequent use of dramatic impersonations (role-playing verbalizations) than did children attending traditional classrooms, even though the classrooms did not differ in total verbal output directed toward peers or teachers. Interestingly, the two types of traditional classrooms did not differ in play level when effects due to ages of children were held constant.

Johnson et al. [1980] observed, for one semester, the free play of 17 children enrolled in a discovery-based preschool and 18 children enrolled in a formal-education preschool program. Although the free play periods in each classroom were similar, formal-education preschoolers attended structured teacher-led small groups where content material was sequentially organized. On the other hand, discovery program preschoolers had additional free play periods. It was found that the formal-program children exhibited significantly more constructive free play than the discovery-program children, who displayed more functional play. Across classrooms, the social level of play and total amount of dramatic play was the same; however, more symbolic transformations during dramatic play were manifested in the formal-education classroom.

Continuing their observations for an additional two semesters, *Johnson and Ershler* [1981] reported that over time formal-program children exhibited less constructive and more dramatic play, while discovery-program children shifted from more functional to more constructive play. These results were considered in relation to differences in program structure. In the formal classroom there was more adult direction in small groups but not during free play. In this classroom children may have found constructive play less attractive as a free play option over time because similar activities were available during small groups. Dramatic play might have increased in this classroom as a possible reaction to the teachers' encouragement for symbolic behavior in the small group sessions. A set for representational behavior may have been carried over into the free play periods. In contrast, teachers in the discovery classroom may have hindered imaginative play development by using free play as a time to teach, albeit by nondidactic methods.

Discussion

Play may be defined as behavior that is intrinsically motivated, freely chosen, process-oriented, and pleasurable. It is also lawful behavior. The search for antecedent conditions of the play of preschool children has led to three general categories of influence. First there is the developmental level of the child. How a child plays depends, in part, on the child's maturational status. For example, pretend play has as one of its prerequisites a certain level of symbolic capability. Second, play expression is a function of individual personality differences and historical antecedents that include the composite effect of cultural and familial determinants. Third, there are situational or context effects. Investigating the contribution of the preschool curriculum to children's play falls into this third category. Understanding curricular effects on play requires identifying mediating variables and mechanisms responsible for them – the specific content, structure, and timing of events within the immediate physical and interpersonal environment as well as relating these variables to developmental and personality characteristics.

Curriculum is a complex multidimensional construct. In this chapter we have highlighted a program structure which was operationalized as the amount of teacher direction and the ratio of convergent to divergent learning activities. This has enabled us to conceptualize a continuum of preschool curricula that served as our framework for examining curricular effects on play. Since the literature evaluating curricular effects on the play of preschoolers has proven to be somewhat limited, the conclusions which follow are based on the empirical research reviewed in this chapter as well as on speculative extrapolations from programs that have not been empirically evaluated.

It appears that highly structured preschools tend to reduce the range, diversity, or maturity level of the play of preschool children [*Beller* et al., 1971; *Huston-Stein* et al., 1977; *Miller and Dyer*, 1975; *Rubin and Seibel*, 1979]. Dramatic and functional play seem to be more common in less structured programs, and constructive or goal-directed manipulative play more common in highly structured programs [*Beller* et al., 1971; *Huston-Stein* et al., 1977; *Johnson and Newman*, 1980; *Miller and Dyer*, 1975; *Rubin*, 1977; *Rubin and Seibel*, 1979]. One might anticipate that dramatic play occurring in more structured programs tends to be more teacher-directed and organized as compared to spontaneous dramatic play commonplace in the less structured programs [*Johnson and Newman*, 1980]. The results of *Tizard* et al. [1976] and *Johnson and Ershler* [1981] may appear inconsistent with the above generalizations. In these comparative studies, it was found that the structured programs were associated with more dramatic play. In both studies, however, the free play of the children did not appear to have been hampered by the structured components of the curriculum. Furthermore, in each case the structured features of the curriculum served to enhance language or representational behavior. Thus, a set of symbolic behavior may have been established that could have positively affected free play behaviors. Second, and more speculatively, it is possible that the content of a program outside of free play may interact with free play to influence preschool play in general [*Johnson and Ershler*, 1981; *Tizard* et al., 1976]. Third, when addressing the question of curricular effects on the play of preschoolers, it is important to distinguish among the different types of play. In most instances, the meaningful questions are what types of preschool play are promoted, discouraged, or ignored by a given curriculum, and how this is accomplished.

Educational Implications

In recent years increased attention has been given to the issues of defining 'good play' and how such forms of play can be increased [*Chance*, 1979]. There appear to be three ways to address these issues. At the risk of oversimplification, these may be referred to as the 'all play is good' response, the 'some types of play are good' response, and the 'all play is not good' response.

The first position generally reflects the views of proponents of the traditional preschool curriculum [*Kleiber*, 1976; *Weininger*, 1979], while the last point of view generally represents the sentiments of those who advocate the 'no-nonsense' or 'back-to-basics' approach to early childhood education. The intermediate position, the one that for over the past 20 years has received increased attention, has been discussed in a variety of ways. For instance, *Gelbach* [1976] distinguished between 'educational play' and 'ordinary play', and *Spodeck* [1974] noted the differences between 'educational play' and 'recreational play'.

Gelbach [1976] considered play educational if the activity incorporated instructional functions normally performed by the teacher. For educational play there needs to be specified incremental learning objectives as well as the provision of practice and discriminative feedback. *Gelbach* [1976] noted that adults can systematically design play equipment and activities to produce predictable results. However, to maintain its status as a play activity it is necessary for the activity to remain player-centered, i.e., initiated, paced, and stylized by the child and not the teacher. *Spodeck* [1974] discussed educational play as activity that includes teacher involvement. Such play has learning consequences unlike recreational play, but again the adult is reminded that too much imposition can disrupt the play activity altogether. Teachers are urged to become more of a play connoisseur and to intervene at opportune moments to raise the level of the child's behavior from a lower level of social or cognitive play to a higher level. If the child is playing to capacity the child presumably is more likely to gain developmentally.

On the other hand, mere teacher's presence or participation does not guarantee that play will be educational. Some play engineered by the teacher may do little more than amuse or entertain the child; some play may bore or frustrate the child. To contribute to the development or education of the child, play opportunities need to be appropriate and challenging. Some play opportunities may tap innovative or divergent problem-solving behaviors, while others may involve conventional or convergent problem-solving behavior. In either case, it ultimately depends on the child whether the activity is educational in the sense of the child acquiring or practicing some skill important to development. Teacher involvement is not even necessary at times.

Others are also becoming more concerned with preschool play. For example, *Goldman and Chaillé* [1981] recommend a more active role of teachers in facilitating creative object use and object use with peers in the preschool. Based upon their systematic observations, they considered object use activities to be an 'underdeveloped resource', especially in child-development-oriented programs that incorporate a strong free play component. In a similar vein, others [*Christie*, 1980; *Rubin*, 1980; *Smith*, 1978] have suggested enriching the free play curriculum by implementing some of the techniques developed in the fantasy play training research. Although additional research is necessary to assess the long-term consequences of fantasy play training and the role of adult tuition, such enriched play may form the basis of an alternative approach to the traditional free play curriculum that has run into sharp criticisms of late [*Tizard*, 1977].

Summary and Speculations

Constructing a diversified play environment that permits a variety of types of play to occur is often viewed as a critical component of the preschool curriculum. Different cognitive, social cognitive, and social skills may be enhanced by including an assortment of play activities and materials available to the child [*Rubin*, 1977; *Sponseller*, 1974]. In addition, variety in play opportunities better serves individual differences that are known to exist among preschoolers in their play predisposition [*Pulaski*, 1970]. *Prescott* [1978] makes the important point that the day-care or preschool curriculum needs to take into account the goodness of fit between the needs of each individual child and what the environment has to offer. This implies the necessity of flexibility in formulating curricula and anticipating outcomes.

Different forms of cognitive and social play may be seen to relate to particular curricular components. Teaching goals based upon the educational philosophy of the program, as well as regional or community differences in the value given to play, give direction to the types of play (such as functional, constructive, or dramatic) that a program may promote; or determine whether play should be promoted at all. Factors that maximize constructive play, for example, would seem to include teacher instruction and encouragement for this type of play, as well as the provision of appropriate materials that match the cognitive and interest levels of the child. On the other hand, minimal amounts of constructive play would be expected when the conditions of the program are distracting, such as when there are too many children, not enough space, minimal adult supervision, or activities and materials that are too advanced for the cognitive capabilities of the children enrolled in the program.

Functional and dramatic play would appear to be more likely in programs that have few constraints on and little evaluation of children's behavior, and when there is enough time given for these forms of play to take place and develop. Dramatic play in particular can be expected to flourish in programs where teachers encourage and model make-believe play and provide a variety of pretend-play props, including structured and representational toys as well as unstructured play materials. A minimum of dramatic play would occur in programs that restrict the time and space necessary for this form of play to occur. In addition, one would expect little pretending in programs with teachers who are disinterested or opposed to make-believe or who inadvertently set out an overabundance of realistic props or single solution toys which are all too obvious and limiting as to their use.

It is very difficult to draw even tentative conclusions regarding the influence of the preschool curriculum on the social level of children's play. Very little research has been done focussing on social play under different preschool curricula. Given the association between parallel and constructive play and between interactive play and functional or dramatic play [*Johnson and Ershler*, 1981; *Rubin*, 1977], one may infer that less structured programs would favor higher levels of social play. High levels of teacher direction may decrease opportunities for peer interactions, and an emphasis on convergent learning may not be as valuable as an emphasis on divergent learning experiences for the development of important social skills. The flexibility of thinking of a variety of responses that is involved in divergent learning may be related to the ability to incorporate another's point of view in a social interaction. *Spivack and Shure* [1974] have reported that the social adjustment of young children is mediated by the ability to think of a number of different responses to social situations.

There are many complex determinants and processes in curricular effects on the play of preschoolers. The greatest obstacle to forming generalizations at this time is the limited empirical data base. In the future, researchers would do well to examine the following issues raised in this chapter:

(1) What is the relationship between proximal antecedent conditions (teacher behavior, play provisions) and the philosophy of a preschool program?

(2) What is the relationship between preexisting characteristics of children and the influence of a given preschool program? That is, can individual difference variables moderate curricular effects on play?

(3) What is the relationship between programming during free play and programming during other times of the school day. That is, we need research on factors that can qualify curricular effects or that interact with components of curricula and thus lead indirectly to differences in children's play.

Finally, although not discussed in this chapter, it would be useful to determine how experience in a preschool program can influence play outside the classroom, such as at home, or can have long-term consequences on play:

(4) What is the relationship between play competence (both social and cognitive) and different preschool curricula?

(5) What is the relationship between play competence and play performance in different preschool curricula?

Needless to say, research addressing itself to any of the above issues would confront considerable conceptual and methodological difficulties. However, such research would lead to a better understanding of the direction and magnitude of curricular effects on the play of young children. As a result, the gap between what is known about curricular effects on cognitive test performance and what is known about curricular effects on play behavior would narrow, thereby improving the state of program evaluation.

References

Ammon, P.R.: Cognitive development and early childhood education: Piagetian and neo-Piagetian theories; in Horn, Robinson, Psychological processes in early education (Academic Press, New York 1977).

Bakeman, R.; Brownlee, J.R.: The strategic use of parallel play: a sequential analysis. Child Dev. *51:* 873–878 (1980).

Beller, E.K.; Zimmie, J.; Aiken, L.: Levels of play in different nursery settings. Int. Congr. Appl. Psychol., Liège 1971.

Bereiter, C.; Engelmann, S.: Teaching disadvantaged children in the preschool (Prentice-Hall, Englewood Cliffs 1966).

Chance, P.: Learning through play (Gardner Press, New York 1979).

Christie, J.F.: Play: to train or not to train? 6th Annu. Meet. Ass. Anthropol. Study of Play, Ann Arbor 1980.

Cupp, J.R.: An instructional program for three- and four-year-old disadvantaged children. Mimeographed. Demonstration and Research Center for Early Education (George Peabody College for Teachers 1967).

Dreyer, A.; Rigler, D.: Cognitive performance in Montessori and nursery school children. J. educ. Res. *62:* 411–416 (1969).

Gelbach, T.: Educational play: a definition for applied research. Annu. Conf. Am. Educ. Res. Ass., San Francisco 1976.

Goldman, J.; Chaillé, C.: Object use in the preschool: an underdeveloped resource. Bien. Meet. Soc. Res. Child Dev., Boston 1981.

Griffing, P.: The relationship between socioeconomic status and sociodramatic play among black kindergarten children. Genet. Psychol. Monogr. *101:* 3–34 (1980).

Hess, R.D.; Croft, D.J.: Teachers of young children (Houghton Mifflin, Boston 1972).

Huston-Stein, A.; Freidrich-Cofer, L.; Susman, E.: The relationship of classroom structure to social behavior, imaginative play, and self-regulation of economically disadvantaged children. Child Dev. *48:* 908–916 (1977).

Johnson, J.E.; Ershler, J.: Developmental trends in preschool play as a function of classroom program and child gender. Child Dev. *52* (in press 1981).

Johnson, J.E.; Ershler, J.; Bell, C.: Play behavior in a discovery-based and a formal education preschool program. Child Dev. *51:* 271–274 (1980).

Johnson, J.E.; Newman, V.: Imaginative play themes and the teacher's role. Offspring *21:* 25–31 (1980).

Kleiber, D.: Playing to learn. Quest *26:* 68–74 (1976).

Miller, L.B.; Dyer, J.L.: Four preschool programs: their dimensions and effects. Monogr. Soc. Res. Child Dev. *40:* serial No. 162 (1975).

Montessori, M.: The Montessori method (Schoeken, New York 1964).

Moore, N.V.; Evertson, C.M.; Brophy, J.E.: Solitary play: some functional reconsiderations. Devl Psychol. *10:* 830–834 (1974).

Parten, M.B.: Social participation among preschool children. J. abnorm. soc. Psychol. *27:* 243–269 (1932).

Phyfe-Perkins, E.: Children's behavior in preschool settings: a review of research concerning the influence of the physical environment; in Katz, Current topics in early childhood education, vol. 3 (Ablex, Norwood 1980).

Piaget, J.: Play, dreams, and imitation in childhood (Norton, New York 1962).

Prescott, E.: Is day care as good as home? Y. Child *i:* 13–19 (1978).

Pulaski, M.A.: Play as a function of toy structure and fantasy predisposition. Child Dev. *41:* 531–537 (1970).

Rainbow Series: Project Head Start (Office of Economic Opportunity, Washington 1965).

Rubin, K.H.: Play behaviors of young children. Y. Child *iii:* 16–24 (1977).

Rubin, K.H. (ed.): Children's play (Jossey-Bass, San Francisco 1980).

Rubin, K.H.; Krasnor, L.R.: Changes in the play behaviors of preschoolers: a short-term longitudinal investigation. Can. J. behav. Sci./Revue can. Sci. Comp. *12:* 278–282 (1980).

Rubin, K.H.; Seibel, C.G.: The effects of ecological setting on the cognitive and social play behaviors of preschoolers. Annu. Meet. Am. Educ. Res. Ass., San Francisco 1979.

Rubin, K.H.; Maioni, T.L.; Hornung, M.: Free play behaviors in middle- and lower-class preschoolers: Parten and Piaget revisited. Child Dev. *47:* 414–419 (1976).

Rubin, K.H.; Watson, K.S.; Jambor, T.W.: Free play behaviors in preschool and kindergarten children. Child Dev. *49:* 534–536 (1978).

Singer, J.L. (ed.): The child's world of make-believe: experimental studies of imaginative play (Wiley, New York 1973).

Smilansky, S.: The effects of sociodramatic play on disadvantaged preschool children (Wiley, New York 1968).

Smith, P.K.: Social and fantasy play in young children; in Tizard, Harvey, Biology of play (Heinemann, London 1977).

Smith, P.K.: A longitudinal study of social participation in preschool children: solitary and parallel play reexamined. Devl Psychol. *14:* 517–523 (1978).

Spivack, G.; Shure, M.B.: Social adjustment of young children: a cognitive approach to solving real-life problems (Jossey-Bass, San Francisco 1974).

Spodeck, B.: The problem of play: educational or recreational?; in Sponseller, Play as a learning medium (National Association for the Education of Young Children, Washington 1974).

Sponseller, D.: A scheme for play and for learning; in Sponseller, Play as a learning medium (National Association for the Education of Young Children, Washington 1974).

Tizard, B.: Play: the child's way of learning?; in Tizard, Harvey, Biology of play (Heinemann, London 1977).

Tizard, B.; Philps, J.; Plewis, I.: Play in preschool centers. II. Effects on play of the child's social class and of the educational orientation of the center. J. Child Psychol. Psychiat. *17:* 265–274 (1976).

Weininger, O.: Play and education: the basic tool for early childhood learning (Thomas, Springfield 1979).

Contr. hum. Dev., vol. 6, pp. 144–153 (Karger, Basel 1982)

Ecological Influences on Children's Play: Issues and Approaches

David Darvill

University of Waterloo, Waterloo, Ont., Canada

'B = f(P E)' [*Lewin*, 1931]

In this chapter I will sidestep two basic and controversial issues in the study of play, its definition and its function [see chapters by *Rubin*, *Vandenberg*, and *Matthews and Matthews*, this volume]. Instead, I will deal primarily with a more visible issue, the structure of children's play. Specifically, I will consider the influence of the environment on the structure of play.

Psychologists have long suggested that the environment can have an important influence on the behavior of people [*Lewin*, 1931]. Indeed, play, however defined, does not take place in a vacuum. The environment in which a child plays, whether literal or figurative, consists of a setting that is populated with objects or others, or both. Recognition of the possibly important effects of this play environment has been generally lacking in studies of the play of young children. For example, many researchers report simply that their studies were conducted during the children's 'free play' period [*Bott*, 1928; *Rosen*, 1974; *Rubin* et al., 1976] without providing any further details of the play setting. Consequently, since much of the research about children's play involves studies conducted in preschool settings, the reader who believes that environmental influences are important in studying any behavior and who wishes to compare findings from various studies has little choice but to assume that all preschools must be the same, i.e., that all preschools have similar physical layouts and are equipped with identical blocks, art supplies, sandboxes, 'Wendy' houses, and so forth. That this is not the case is intuitively obvious. How then is one to make sensible comparisons of studies of children's play, studies conducted in settings that are seldom the same? Given the necessity of making the aforementioned assumption, without reason to believe that it is valid, perhaps such comparisons are not possible at this time.

If, however, you take the position that there is an obvious and important interaction between the playing child and the physical and social environment, then it is imperative that the environment be well defined before you can determine causes for similarities or differences in children's play that are due to independent variables such as age, sex or different preschool programs. Comparing the results of studies of children's play conducted in different environments must be done with caution, if it can be done at all. In this chapter, therefore, I will briefly outline some issues that may influence this reciprocal relation between children's play behavior and their environment – issues that researchers ought to be aware of when designing and reporting studies of children's play.

What Would Be a Useful Model for Studying Play and Ecology?

Jaynes [1976; p. 53[1]] has suggested that there are differences between models and theories. He gives the following example of the relation between model and theory to illustrate this point: 'A theory is a relationship of the model to the things the model is supposed to represent. The Bohr model of the atom is that of a proton surrounded by orbiting electrons . . . Bohr's *theory* was that all atoms were similar to his *model*. The theory . . . has turned out not to be true. But the model remains. A model is neither true nor false; only the theory of its similarity to what it represents. A theory is thus a metaphor between a model and data.'

To illustrate further, consider the following examples of this relation between model and theory as it applies to the study of play. The first example is based on a model of cognitive growth posited by *Piaget*. This cognitive model had been well developed by *Piaget* and his collaborators over many years [*Flavell*, 1963; *Gruber and Voneche*, 1977]. It is little wonder, therefore, that when *Piaget* [1962] turned to study the development of play the model that he chose was very similar to that which he had developed for cognitive growth. This model of play development included many of the same concepts that were integral to his model of cognitive development, e.g., concepts such as stages, equilibrium, assimilation and accommodation. *Piaget's* [1962] theoretical position on the development of play thus was based on a 'strong'

[1] From The Origins of Consciousness in the Breakdown of the Bicameral Mind by Julian Jaynes. Copyright © 1976 by Julian Jaynes. Reprinted by permission of Houghton Mifflin Company.

model, although the original *data* used to support his theory were based primarily on observations of the play behavior of a very few children (mainly *Piaget's* own 3 children!) and were therefore quite 'weak'. (The data base supporting *Piaget's* model of play, however, has since been greatly expanded by others who have utilized his model and theory.) The types of play behavior posited by *Piaget*, i.e., functional, constructive, symbolic, and games-with-rules, were strongly linked theoretically to this model of play development. They were, however, rather vague with respect to the actual behaviors that each type might encompass, leading to methodological problems that will be discussed below.

Another example of the relation between model and theory in play development involves an ethologically oriented approach to the study of play that is essentially the antithesis of the first example. This approach utilizes a 'strong' *data* base obtained from numerous observational studies involving large numbers of children [*Blurton Jones*, 1972; *McGrew*, 1972a; *Smith and Connolly*, 1972, 1980], but rather 'weak' *models* based primarily on those developed from ethological studies of animal behavior, e.g., models of affiliative relations, dominance hierarchies, aggressive displays and fixed action patterns. In general, the theoretical relations between these 'weak' models and the development of play have also been quite weak. An example of this weakness would be the difficulty of relating specific behaviors or groups of behaviors, e.g., rough-and-tumble play, to any specific developmental theory of play. (The usefulness of these two approaches to the study of play for the derivation of categories of play behavior will be discussed below.)

Neither the Piagetian model of play development nor the ethological models mentioned above, however, include more than a cursory treatment of the effects of the environment on the play behavior of young children. Given our current concern for establishing ecological influences on children's play, what, then, might be an appropriate model for the relation between children's play behavior and the setting in which their behavior takes place?

Fortunately, such a model relating play behavior and environmental factors is not difficult to construct. Foreshadowing the work of later ecological psychologists [*Barker*, 1968; *Barker and Wright*, 1951], *Lewin* [1931, 1936] proposed a 'general law' to govern the relationships among a person, the environment, and the behavior of the person. *Lewin* [1931, 1936] asserted that all behavior (B) is a function of the relationship between the person (P) and the environment (E) or, in quasi-mathematical terms, B = f(P E). He intended that this 'general law' would be valid for any particular dynamic situation and that, as such, it would be applicable to the study of any behavior.

If, therefore, one were to take *Lewin's* 'general law' to be a model of relations among a person, the behavior of that person, and the environment in which the behavior takes place, one could readily modify this model to produce a model of play behavior. Such a modification could be made by specifically concentrating on play behaviors (Bp), the playing child (Pc), and the play setting (Ep). *Lewin's* 'general law' is thus transformed into a 'specific model' wherein a child's play behavior is a function of the relation between the playing child and the play environment. Once again, in quasi-mathematical terms this model becomes Bp = f(Pc Ep). Given such a model, what is then required is to integrate existing models of play, which generally ignore environmental effects on play behavior, into this proposed model, a model that does include the contributions of both personal attributes and environmental attributes as they affect play behavior. Such an integration, however, is beyond the scope of the present chapter. Instead, consider the following points about the proposed model.

Bp=f(Pc Ep)

Most studies of children's play could be catalogued according to a taxonomy based on the three components of the proposed model. For example, there are studies involving the evaluation of changes in children's play behavior (Bp) due to changes or differences in the attributes of the children involved in the study (Pc), e.g., research evaluating the effects on play behavior when children of different ages play in any setting [*Blurton Jones*, 1972; *Smith and Connolly*, 1972]. There are also studies involving an evaluation of the play behaviors of children in different play environments (Ep), e.g., research evaluating the play of the same group of children in different settings [*Smith and Connolly*, 1980]. In addition, another type of study based on this model is also possible. This latter type of study would involve an evaluation of the effects on children's play due to an *interaction* of different children in different play settings and, as such, would require the addition of an interaction term (i.e., Pc Ep) to the proposed model.

Although this proposed model of the relations among play behavior, the playing child, and the play setting appears to be quite simple, this appearance of simplicity belies the complexity of each of the main components of the model. Let us now briefly examine some important aspects of these three components of the proposed model: play behaviors, child attributes, and environmental attributes.

Play Behaviors (Bp)

Recent studies of children's play behavior have typically used one of two very different approaches to determine the categories of behavior that are to be characterized as play. One approach utilizes broad play categories, such as functional, constructive or symbolic play, derived from theoretical suppositions about the ontogenesis of play behavior in young children [*Rosen*, 1974; *Rubin*, 1977a; *Rubin* et al., 1976; *Smilansky*, 1968]. The other approach is ethological in nature and most often involves much narrower categories of behavior, such as climbing or rough-and-tumble play, derived primarily from the actual behaviors of children [*Blurton Jones*, 1972; *Hughes*, 1978; *McGrew*, 1972a; *Smith and Connolly*, 1980].

Consider further the first approach. Many studies of the play behavior of preschool children have dealt with the influence of independent measures such as age or sex on rather broad model-derived categories of play, e.g., cognitive categories such as functional, constructive, and dramatic play [*Piaget*, 1962; *Smilansky*, 1968] or social participation categories such as solitary, parallel, and group play [*Parten*, 1932; *Rubin* et al., 1976]. The results of research using these broad categories have suggested, for example, the developmental sequence of such play categories, i.e., researchers have indicated those play behaviors that are most prominent at particular ages [*Barnes*, 1971; *Parten*, 1932; *Rubin* et al., 1976; *Smilansky*, 1968]. In addition, broad play categories have also been used in studies to evaluate the effects of various environmental factors on children's play. Researchers utilizing such broad categories have attempted to establish how the availability of various toys [*Rubin*, 1977b; *Van Alstyne*, 1932] or the establishment of different areas within a preschool [*Shure*, 1963] can influence children's play behavior.

These broad categories of play, however, are not used without problems. *Bott* [1928, p. 73] for example, attempted to use 'classical distinctions' such as 'manipulative' and 'constructive' to classify the play materials used in a study of children's play activities. She found that 'too often . . . the line between these was hard to draw'. As an illustration of this difficulty, *Bott* [1928] presented the following case. The youngest, 2-year-old children in her study played with a toy called a 'tinker builder' in a rather casual way. The 3-year-old children, however, used this same toy in a constructive fashion, whereas the oldest children, from 4 to 5 years old, created complex figures with the tinker builder. Thus the tinker builder was used by the children in different ways at different ages, leading to difficulty in classifying the toy as manipulative or constructive with respect to the type of play behavior associated with its use.

Now, consider the second approach to the study of children's play. Recently, ethologists have conducted observational studies of the play behavior of preschool-aged children using time sampling techniques. *Blurton Jones* [1972] traced changes with age in the interactions between children by observing the frequency of narrow categories of behavior such as take, grab-tug, wrestle, jump, paint, etc. *Smith and Connolly* [1972] used similar observational methods and categories of behavior to assess the patterns of play and social interaction in the behavior of preschool-aged children. Aspects of the environment that have been studied with respect to these narrow categories of behavior include, among others, two dimensions of crowding, i.e., social density or the number of persons in a given area [*McGrew*, 1972a; *Smith and Connolly*, 1980] and spatial density or the area per person, and the quantity of play resources available to the children [see *Phyfe-Perkins*, 1980; *Smith and Connolly*, 1980, for recent reviews]. These ethological studies have dealt mainly with social aspects of children's play such as the amount of rough-and-tumble play, the amount of group play, and the effects of crowding [*Blurton Jones*, 1972; *Roper and Hinde*, 1978; *Smith*, 1977; *Smith and Connolly*, 1972, 1980], possibly because social behaviors are easier to observe in a preschool setting than are cognitive activities.

The results of research involving both of the above approaches, the one using broad categories of play behavior derived mainly from play models and the other using narrow categories and patterns of play primarily derived from children's actual behaviors, have been generally consistent in painting a picture of the development of the 'free play' behaviors of preschool-aged children, i.e., the type of play that can be expected at a particular age and how the various types of play change with age. Furthermore, both approaches have been useful in establishing some effects of the environment on various aspects of children's play, as previously mentioned.

There are, however, several problems associated with these two approaches to the study of play. In the first case, there is an inherent vagueness in the definitions of the broad, model-based cognitive categories of play [*Bott*, 1928], e.g., dramatic play is defined as 'the substitution of an imaginary situation to satisfy the child's personal wishes and needs' [*Rubin*, 1977a; see *Matthews and Matthews*, this volume, for an interesting discussion of and possible solution to this problem with respect to fantasy play]. In addition, the broad cognitive categories are not mutually exclusive with respect to each other. There is, for example, an implied hierarchy among the cognitive categories of play such that 'dramatic' play may include 'constructive' or 'functional' activities, or both, but neither 'constructive' nor 'functional' play can include 'dramatic' activities.

In the second case, many of the behavior categories used in the ethological studies are so specifically defined as to be of questionable value in the study of play development, e.g., 'play beat' is defined as a 'sharp downward movement of hand towards another child, usually from above shoulder level; no physical contact or agonism' [*Smith and Connolly*, 1980]. It is perhaps apparent from the labelling of this example as 'play' beat that more than simply the behavior is implied in the definition. One must usually have some knowledge of the context in which the behavior occurs as well as some a priori definition of play in order to establish that an observed behavior is indeed playful and not simply a missed agonistic hit. *Smith and Connolly* [1972] considered this need for a 'situation analysis' of the context of the behavior to be a reservation concerning the ethological approach. *Matthews and Matthews* [this volume], however, make use of the implicit, a priori definition of play that most people have by asking observers to rate children's behavior as fantasy play if it meets the criterion that 'that is a case of fantasy if anything'. Perhaps recognizing these problems, some ethologists who have used specific behavioral definitions have also included forms of the 'vague' categories of play [*Blurton Jones*, 1972; *Smith and Connolly*, 1980]. *Smith and Connolly* [1972] have perhaps carried this latter approach to an extreme by using only one category of play, labelled simply 'play'.

As can be ascertained from the above discussion, choosing appropriate categories of play for any study is no simple task; some categories are too vague or broadly defined, whereas others are too narrowly defined. Needless to say, the choice of behaviors to be studied should be bound to the question that is to be asked; there are no 'correct' categories of play behavior, only 'appropriate to the question' categories.

Child Attributes (Pc)

The *history* of a child within the particular setting of a study obviously will have an effect on the child's behavior in that setting. *George Santayana* succinctly noted that 'the same battle in the clouds will be known to the deaf only as lightning and to the blind only as thunder'. When a child is in an unfamiliar setting, for example, the probability of exploratory behaviors by the child increases prior to the beginning of any play in the setting [*Berlyne*, 1966; *Hughes*, 1978; *Hutt*, 1979].

In addition, the *relationships* of a 'focal' child to the others in the setting will also have an effect on the focal child's behavior. *McGrew* [1972b], for instance, found children to be subdued and exhibit signs of ambivalence when first introduced to an unfamiliar preschool group. Several recent studies have also contrasted the play behavior of acquainted versus non-acquainted partners [*Doyle* et al., 1980; *Gottman and Parkhurst*, 1978]. *Doyle* et al. [1980] found, for example, that sustained fantasy play occurred more often with familiar playmates than with unfamiliar playmates. Their findings and those of others [*Krasnor and Darvill*, 1980] suggest that the affiliative relationships of the 'focal' child with the others in his or her group may be an important variable influencing the child's play within a setting. Also of possible importance in this respect is the 'focal' child's position in the dominance hierarchy of a group [*Sluckin and Smith*, 1977; *Strayer and Strayer*, 1976] since, in animal studies, more dominant animals have been shown to have greater access to the available resources in a setting [*Hausfater*, 1975; *Kummer*, 1971].

Environmental Attributes (Ep)

Any environment can be viewed from at least two broad perspectives, molecular and molar [*Lewin*, 1936]. On the one hand, children's play will be affected by *molecular* dimensions of the environment. These molecular dimensions include those aspects of the environment that are readily discernable by the child, e.g., toys and other play equipment or other people, such as peers, other-aged children or adults. In addition, there are other aspects of the molecular environment that are less recognizable by the child, e.g., the spatial density, social density, or sex ratio of the children in the play area.

On the other hand, *molar* dimensions of the environment can also affect the play of a child, dimensions such as the socioeconomic status of the child's family [*Smilansky*, 1968] or the general cultural norms concerned with the play of children [*Schwartzman*, 1978]. As an example of such molar effects, studies comparing the play behavior of children from families of different socioeconomic status have found that the play of lower socioeconomic status children involves quantitatively and qualitatively lower levels of sociodramatic or fantasy play compared to the play of higher socioeconomic status children. It has been suggested that differences in the home environments of these two groups may be one reason for these differences in play behavior [*Rosen*, 1974; *Smilansky*, 1968].

In any case, researchers should be aware of the multidimensional nature of the environment in which children live and play. Researchers must not only consider the effects on a child's play of the actual setting in which the child's play behavior is observed, but also be aware of possible effects of the environment beyond the immediate play setting.

One would do well to keep in mind that there is 'no limit on variables one could include in analysis of any theory – (the) crucial task is to pick the right variable' [*Arbib*, 1972, p. 58]. In trying to assess the complex influences of the environment on children's play, there are a great many potentially important variables to be examined before the complete story is known.

as I am looking at culture, putting both cultures in a semi-structured but still natural environment is controlling one of two major variables

References

Arbib, M.A.: The metaphorical brain (Wiley, New York 1972).

Barker, R.G.: Ecological psychology (Stanford University Press, Stanford 1968).

Barker, R.G.; Wright, H.F.: One boy's day (Harper & Row, New York 1951).

Barnes, K.: Preschool play norms: a replication. Devl Psychol. *5:* 99–103 (1971).

Berlyne, D.E.: Curiosity and exploration. Science *153:* 25–33 (1966).

Blurton Jones, N.: Categories of child-child interaction; in Blurton Jones, Ethological studies of child behavior (Cambridge University Press, Cambridge 1972).

Bott, H.: Observation of play activities in a nursery school. Genet. Psychol. Monogr. *4:* 44–88 (1928).

Doyle, A.B.; Connolly, J.; Rivest, L.: The effect of playmate familiarity on social interactions of young children. Child Dev. *51:* 217–223 (1980).

Flavell, J.: The developmental psychology of Jean Piaget (Van Nostrand & Reinhold, New York 1963).

Gottman, J.; Parkhurst, J.: A developmental theory of friendship and acquaintanceship process. Minnesota Symp. on Child Psychol., 1978.

Gruber, H.E.; Voneche, J.J.: The essential Piaget (Basic Books, New York 1977).

Hausfater, G.: Dominance and reproduction in baboons *(Papio cynocephalus):* a quantitative analysis. Contr. Primatol., vol. 7 (Karger, Basel 1975).

Hughes, M.: Sequential analysis of exploration and play. Int. J. Behav. Dev. *1:* 83–97 (1978).

Hutt, C.: Exploration and play; in Sutton-Smith, Play and learning (Gardner, New York 1979).

Jaynes, J.: The origin of consciousness in the breakdown of the bicameral mind (University of Toronto Press, Toronto 1976).

Krasnor, L.R.; Darvill, D.: Friendship and play: effects of companions on the structure of play. University of Waterloo Conf. on Child Dev., 1980.

Kummer, H.: Primate societies: group techniques of ecological adaptation (Aldine, Chicago 1971).

Lewin, K.: Environmental forces in child behavior and development; in Murchison, A handbook of child psychology (Clark University Press, Worcester 1931).

Lewin, K.: Principles of topological psychology (McGraw-Hill, New York 1936).

McGrew, W.C.: An ethological study of children's play (Academic Press, New York 1972a).

McGrew, W.C.: Aspects of social development in nursery school children, with emphasis on introduction to the group; in Blurton Jones, Ethological studies of child behavior (Cambridge University Press, Cambridge 1972b).

Parten, M.B.: Social participation among preschool children. J. abnorm. soc. Psychol. *27:* 243–269 (1932).

Phyfe-Perkins, E.: Children's behavior in preschool settings. A review of research concerning the influence of the physical environment; in Katz, Current topics in early childhood education, vol. 3 (Ablex, Norwood N.J. 1980).

Piaget, J.: Play, dreams, and imitation (Norton, New York 1962).

Roper, R.; Hinde, R.A.: Social behavior in a play group: consistency and complexity. Child Dev. *49:* 570–579 (1978).

Rosen, C.E.: The effects of sociodramatic play on problem solving behavior among culturally disadvantaged children. Child Dev. *45:* 920–927 (1974).

Rubin, K.H.: The behaviors of young children. Young Children *32:* 16–24 (1977a).

Rubin, K.H.: The social and cognitive value of preschool toys and activities. Can. J. behav. Sci. *9:* 382–385 (1977b).

Rubin, K.H.; Maioni, T.L.; Hornung, M.: Free play behaviors in middle and lower class preschoolers: Parten and Piaget revisited. Child Dev. *47:* 414–419 (1976).

Schwartzman, H.B.: Transformations: the anthropology of children's play (Plenum, New York 1978).

Shure, M.E.: Psychological ecology of a nursery school. Child Dev. *34:* 979–994 (1963).

Sluckin, A.M.; Smith, P.K.: Two approaches to the concept of dominance in preschool children. Child Dev. *48:* 917–923 (1977).

Smilansky, S.: The effects of sociodramatic play on disadvantaged preschool children (Wiley, New York 1968).

Smith, P.K.: Social and fantasy play in young children; in Tizard, Harvey, Biology of play (Heinemann, London 1977).

Smith, P.K.; Connolly, K.: Patterns of play and social interaction in pre-school children; in Blurton Jones, Ethological studies of child behavior (Cambridge University Press, Cambridge 1972).

Smith, P.K.; Connolly, K.: The ecology of preschool behavior (Cambridge University Press, Cambridge 1980).

Strayer, F.F.; Strayer, J.: An ethological analysis of social agonism and dominance relations among preschool children. Child Dev. *47:* 980–989 (1976).

Van Alstyne, D.: Play behavior and choice of play materials of preschool children (University of Chicago Press, Chicago 1932).

Biographical Sketches

Debra J. Pepler is a research associate in psychology at the Centre for Research in Human Development, Erindale College, University of Toronto. Her research interests include the relationship of play and divergent and convergent problem-solving, and sibling interaction.

Kenneth H. Rubin is professor of developmental psychology at the University of Waterloo. His research interests include communicative, social, and social-cognitive development in young children. He has authored, co-authored or edited three books and numerous chapters and journal articles. He is currently an Associate Editor of *Child Development*.

Author Index